Teaching **Yoga** for Life

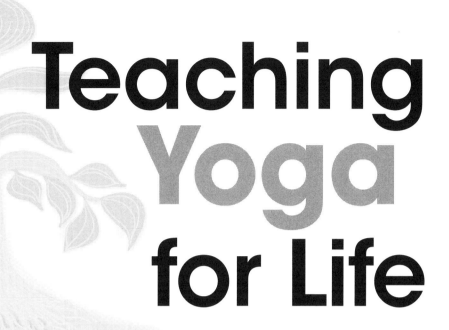

Teaching Yoga for Life

Preparing Children and Teens for Healthy, Balanced Living

Nanette E. Tummers, EdD

Eastern Connecticut State University

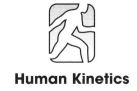

Human Kinetics

Library of Congress Cataloging-in-Publication Data

Tummers, Nanette.
    Teaching yoga for life : preparing children and teens for healthy, balanced living / Nanette Tummers.
       p. cm.
    Includes bibliographical references.
    ISBN-13: 978-0-7360-7016-4 (softcover)
    ISBN-10: 0-7360-7016-8 (softcover)
    1. Hatha yoga for children--Study and teaching. 2. Hatha yoga for teenagers--Study and teaching. I. Title.
    RJ133.7.T86 2009
    613.7'046083--dc22

                                   2008029011

ISBN-10: 0-7360-7016-8
ISBN-13: 978-0-7360-7016-4

Acquisitions Editor: Gayle Kassing, PhD
Developmental Editor: Ragen E. Sanner
Assistant Editor: Anne Rumery
Copyeditor: Patricia MacDonald
Proofreader: Joanna Hatzopoulos Portman
Permission Manager: Dalene Reeder
Graphic Designer: Robert Reuther
Graphic Artist: Patrick Sandberg
Cover Designer: Keith Blomberg
Photographer (cover and interior): Neil Bernstein, unless otherwise noted
Photo Asset Manager: Laura Fitch
Photo Production Manager: Jason Allen
Art Manager: Kelly Hendren
Associate Art Manager: Alan L. Wilborn
Illustrator: Mic Greenberg
Printer: Edwards Brothers

Printed in the United States of America   10 9 8 7 6 5 4 3 2 1

Human Kinetics
Web site: www.HumanKinetics.com

United States: Human Kinetics
P.O. Box 5076
Champaign, IL 61825-5076
800-747-4457
e-mail: humank@hkusa.com

Canada: Human Kinetics
475 Devonshire Road Unit 100
Windsor, ON N8Y 2L5
800-465-7301 (in Canada only)
e-mail: info@hkcanada.com

Europe: Human Kinetics
107 Bradford Road
Stanningley
Leeds LS28 6AT, United Kingdom
+44 (0) 113 255 5665
e-mail: hk@hkeurope.com

Australia: Human Kinetics
57A Price Avenue
Lower Mitcham, South Australia 5062
08 8372 0999
e-mail: info@hkaustralia.com

New Zealand: Human Kinetics
Division of Sports Distributors NZ Ltd.
P.O. Box 300 226 Albany
North Shore City
Auckland
0064 9 448 1207
e-mail: info@humankinetics.co.nz

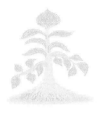

This book is dedicated to my true yoga teachers: my family, friends, colleagues, and students.

Contents

Activity Finder

Title	Page	Type of pose or activity
Action story	77	Indoor Recess
"As If" game	77	Indoor Recess
Morning routine	78	Indoor Recess
Balloon breath, three-part breath, yoga breath, or Dirga breath	85	Breath
Belly breath	87	Breath
Bunny nose, whale spout breath, or dragon breath	88	Breath
Green meanies	88	Breath
Heart breath	89	Breath
Hummingbird breath or buzzing bee breath	89	Breath
Lion's roar	90	Breath
Peace train	90	Breath
Quieting breath or chilling breath	91	Breath
Release and recharge breath or R & R breath	91	Breath
Alternate nostril breathing	92	Breathing exercise for older students
Ujjayi breath, Darth Vader, or ocean-sounding breath	92	Breathing exercise for older students
Beach balls	94	Relaxation
Chair relaxation	94	Relaxation
Child pose	95	Relaxation
Hammock	95	Relaxation
Kermit the Frog	96	Relaxation
Legs up against the wall	96	Relaxation
Lying gentle spine-twist pose or angels in the snow	97	Relaxation
Macaroni test	98	Relaxation
Meltdown	98	Relaxation
Nose to knees, hugs, or bug in a rug	99	Relaxation
Relaxation pose, Shavasana, quiet pose, or Sleeping Beauty	100	Relaxation
Volcano	101	Relaxation
Color me peaceful	102	Visualization

Title	Page	Type of pose or activity
Sun, moon, and star dance	135	Moving yoga
Sunflower and cactus dance	135	Moving yoga
Arrow	136	Balancing pose
Eagle or noodle	136	Balancing pose
Lighthouse	137	Balancing pose, grades 5+
Standing bow, flamingo, stork, or dancer	137	Balancing pose, grades 3+
Tree	138	Balancing pose
Warrior III, T pose, or airplane	138	Balancing pose
Boat	140	Active floor pose
Bridge	141	Active floor pose
Kneeling back-bend pose or camel	142	Active floor pose
Lying-down bow	142	Active floor pose
Plank, pirate's plank, or push-up	143	Active floor pose
Reverse plank or slide	143	Active floor pose
Ride a bike	144	Active floor pose, grades pre-K-3
Shark	145	Active floor pose
Side plank or rainbow	145	Active floor pose, grades 5+
Superhero	146	Active floor pose
Butterfly	148	Cool-down pose
Fetal or reflection pose	149	Cool-down pose
Happy baby	149	Cool-down pose
Seated straight-leg forward fold	150	Cool-down pose
Seated twist	151	Cool-down pose
Turtle	152	Cool-down pose
Windshield wipers	153	Cool-down pose
Chime time	157	Yoga game for younger students
Crazy frogs	157	Yoga game for younger students
Dogs in a row	157	Yoga game for younger students
Driving the car	158	Yoga game for younger students
Elephant, elephant—leader of the jungle	158	Yoga game for younger students
Roller coaster	158	Yoga game for younger students
Oodles of noodles	159	Yoga game
Red light, green light	160	Yoga game
Robot doing yoga	161	Yoga game
Twelve days of yoga	161	Yoga game
Yogi says	161	Yoga game

Title	Page	Type of pose or activity
Color my breathing	179	Art
Trace a pose	179	Art
Yoga T-shirt	179	Art
Making art for others	180	Art for older students
Shell necklace or bracelet and poses on the beach	181	Art for older students
Alphabet soup and learning letters	181	Literacy for younger students
Make up a rhyme	181	Literacy for younger students
Everyday warriors	182	Literacy
I am a mountain	182	Literacy
State, national, or world geography	182	Literacy
Relaxation scripts	182	Literacy for older students
The Berenstain Bears on the Moon	183	Books
Dr. Seuss' *My Many Colored Days*	184	Books
Exploring my environment	184	Science
The farm	184	Science
Nature and yoga poses	184	Science
Bridge and triangle poses	185	Science for older students

Pose Index

Title	Page	Type of pose	Photo
POSES			
Arrow	136	Balancing pose	Photo courtesy of Gregory Kane.
Boat	140	Active floor pose	
Bridge	141	Active floor pose	
Butterfly	148	Cool-down pose	

Title	Page	Type of pose	Photo
Eagle or noodle	136	Balancing pose	
Elephant	122	Standing pose	
Extended side angle or super side stretch	123	Standing pose	

Photo courtesy of Sara Gustavesen.

Title	Page	Type of pose	Photo
Lying-down bow	142	Active floor pose	
Mountain	124	Standing pose	
Plank, pirate's plank, or push-up	143	Active floor pose	
Quarter moon, crescent moon, lateral flexion, or side bend	125	Standing pose	

Title	Page	Type of pose	Photo
Reverse plank or slide	143	Active floor pose	
Ride a bike	144	Active floor pose, grades pre-K-3	Photo courtesy of Gregory Kane
Rock the baby	112	Warm-up	
Rocket ship	126	Standing pose	
Runner's lunge	127	Standing pose	

Title	Page	Type of pose	Photo
Seated straight-leg forward fold	150	Cool-down pose	
Seated twist	151	Cool-down pose	
Shake it up	117	Moving warm-up	
Shark	145	Active floor pose	

Title	Page	Type of pose	Photo
Side plank or rainbow	145	Active floor pose, grades 5+	
Soaking-wet dog	118	Moving warm-up	
Standing back bend or back extension	127	Standing pose	

Title	Page	Type of pose	Photo
Standing bow, flamingo, stork, or dancer	137	Balancing pose, grades 3+	
Standing forward fold, rag doll, or Jell-O melt	128	Standing pose	
Standing frog into squat	119	Moving warm-up	
Standing twisters or blenders	120	Moving warm-up	

Title	Page	Type of pose	Photo
Standing wide-angle forward fold	129	Standing pose	
Superhero	146	Active floor pose	
Table with cow and cat	112	Warm-up	
Tipping star	130	Standing pose	
Tree	138	Balancing pose	

Title	Page	Type of pose	Photo
Triangle	130	Standing pose	
Turning tops	114	Warm-up	
Turtle	152	Cool-down pose	
Upward-facing dog, or up dog	115	Warm-up	
Warrior III, T pose, or airplane	138	Balancing pose	

Title	Page	Type of pose	Photo
Warriors	131	Standing pose	
Windshield wipers	153	Cool-down pose	Photo courtesy of Gregory Kane
Yoga jumping jacks	116	Warm-up	
SUN SALUTATIONS			
Silly wiggle sun dance	134	Moving yoga, pre-K-2	

Title	Page	Type of pose	Photo
Sun dance	134	Moving yoga	
Sun, moon, and star dance	135	Moving yoga	
Sunflower and cactus dance	135	Moving yoga	

Preface

It is difficult to compete with all the distractions young people face: the bells, whistles, and lights of electronics and technology that have captured the attention and energy of our youth. More and more students are turning away from activity and tuning into MP3 and DVD players. How can we provide activity that engages students in meaningful, challenging, and fun ways? With the ever-increasing technological mentality that society is pressuring us to assume, yoga helps us take a step back and discover a renewal of energy within that encourages healthy and balanced living.

Yoga is research based and experiential. It encourages multiple intelligences to engage all of our students, especially students who do not enjoy traditional sports-based activities. Yoga's numerous benefits include improving life skills such as self-awareness and emotional intelligence and developing character and responsibility. Yoga has been around for thousands of years because it works, and it is critically needed now.

Yoga doesn't require the teacher or the students to be experts or to compete with each other. It simply requires a willingness to participate and be open. Yoga is inclusive because it can be adapted to benefit all participants. It can provide a safe and calming atmosphere for students and requires little or no equipment or space.

PURPOSE OF THE BOOK

The purpose of this book is to provide a resource for integrating yoga into an existing physical education class or curriculum (e.g., indoor recess in a classroom, a stressless break in the classroom or cafeteria) or as a stand-alone class (e.g., physical education or teen yoga at a recreation center). This book provides an effective and practical approach to teaching yoga based on National Association for Sport and Physical Education (NASPE) pedagogical standards. The curriculum includes basic physical poses, breathing techniques, relaxation methods, kinesthetic play, and visualizations. The information provided is based on applied research and evidence from piloted programs.

SIGNIFICANCE OF THE BOOK

Teaching Yoga for Life will help the reader understand the inclusive nature of yoga: that anyone can do it. Yoga allows for an experiential model of learning that stresses the importance of individuality. Not many activities that we provide for students allow for this.

Yoga has been gaining more and more momentum as a physical activity in the West and should be viewed as a healthy and balanced living teaching system that not only provides physical activity but also includes mental, emotional, social, and spiritual aspects. Equally important is the emerging acceptance of yoga within the scientific community. The National Institutes of Health (NIH) has a division titled the National Center for Complementary and Alternative Medicine (NCCAM). Numerous studies have explored the efficacy of yoga and its effect on health. We are witnessing yoga gaining popularity in hospitals, corporations, prisons, military bases, universities, and community settings.

Included in this book is a brief introduction to yoga philosophy in simplified "take-home messages" about how to live a better life. It is important that yoga teachers focus not only on the physical exercise but also on a healthy and balanced model of living. It is a mind–body activity that can be practiced for a lifetime.

Parents and school districts may have the mistaken impression that yoga is a religious practice. Yoga may be marginalized because of these misconceptions. *Teaching Yoga for Life* provides the reader with numerous insights as to why yoga is vital in the lives of students. The emphasis of this text is on how yoga can enrich student health in a developmentally sound way. The book provides instruction to safely teach yoga in the context of a lifelong healthy and balanced living practice and with a pedagogical emphasis.

This book honors that the reader is a teacher, has some background in movement, and has a willingness and passion to provide experiential activities for students (e.g., student-centered learning) and a belief in the importance of quality activity for healthy and balanced living. Yoga honors the natural teacher in all of us that comes only with experience, even when many of us who have been teaching physical activity may think, *Been there and taught that.* Yoga is a wonderful way to explore these gifts of teaching even further!

Acknowledgments

I would like to thank Gayle Kassing, Ragen Sanner, and Anne Rumery for their amazing work, guidance, and patience. Human Kinetics is an amazing publisher and company and I appreciate all they have done to make this book happen.

I would also like to thank all of my yoga and wellness teachers who have shared their wealth of experience and knowledge. I would like to express heartfelt gratitude to Mr. Parsons and the University of Miami Wellness Center where I started teaching yoga to older adults and athletes and many thanks to ECSU and my department colleagues for their unwavering support.

Many thanks are also due to the numerous students that allowed me to share the gift of yoga: McSweeny Senior Center; Next Step Perception House; Connecticut Center for Addiction Recovery; Connecticut College; Mansfield and Willimantic school districts; Eastern Connecticut State University, including the HPE department, ECSU baseball team, and the Early Childhood Development Center; Camp Horizons; Mansfield Community Center; the Connecticut chapter of the American Association of Health, Physical Education and Recreation; and Journey House.

Thank you to my family: my parents Jeff and Liesje, my sister Jessica, and my brother Nick. I need to thank my two creative directors: my nephew Justin Tummers Flavell who was both a model and artist for this book and nephew Lucas James Flavell who was a photographer. A sincere thank you to my dear friend, Leslie Clark, for her guidance concerning working with very young children. Thank you to my mentee Sara Gustavesen, for your friendship, enthusiasm, and providing photos of your nieces and nephews Matthew Tiffany, Haley Tiffany, Lydia Tourtellotte, and Alison Tourtellotte. Thank you to Mollie Desjarlais and Stephanie Norell—wonderful models. Thank you to the models at Human Kinetics—Molly Blazier, Iain Carpenter, Trinity Carpenter, Andrew Cribbett, Elise Ellinger, Becky Ramos, Estella Samii, and Nicholas White—you were a joy to work with!

Finally, thank you, Gomez, Augustus, and Lucy—yoga is a natural part of your canine days—thanks for letting me hang with you.

chapter 1

Why Our Students Need Yoga

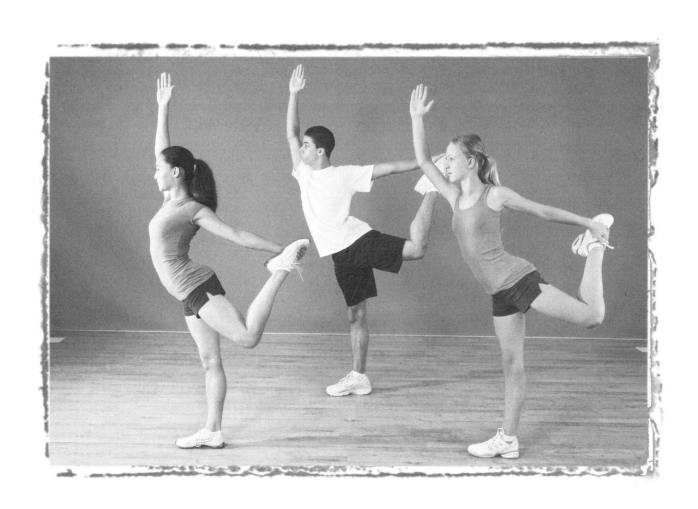

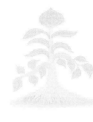

Yoga has multiple definitions and images in Western culture. It may be assumed yoga is synonymous with images of slim bodies contorting into impossible pretzel-like poses; sweaty, exhaustive workouts; strange chanting in a trancelike state; or the ultradisciplined religious practice of yoga gurus. Our frenetic culture's tendency to spin yoga into the latest and greatest fitness fad does not reflect its essential spirit and intention.

What makes yoga different from stretching or working out is yoga's unique ability to connect the body, spirit, and mind inward. Yoga originates from the Sanskrit meaning "to yoke," to bring together the mind, sprit, and body. The inward focus allows for reflection and getting in touch with feelings, emotions, and what is going on in the body. This intention of yoga is to maximize your potential and to embrace the interconnectedness of the spirit, mind, and body.

Our youth have more knowledge and access to the world but seem to have little knowledge of their own bodies and minds. Spend a few minutes observing the youth of today in shopping malls, in school yards, and in the news, and it will not take long to realize that the United States is a nation at risk—severe risk. Among our students are unprecedented rates of obesity, learning issues, bullying, school violence, stress, and depression (www.cdc.gov/mmwr/PDF/SS/SS5505.pdf). For the first time in history, the current generation is not expected to live as long or have the quality of life of their parents' generation if we continue with the status quo.

Yoga offers a way for our students to reconnect with their bodies and minds and become healthy, responsible, and productive participants in society. Foremost in its benefits, yoga provides a safe and nurturing environment for fostering physical, psychological, intellectual, and spiritual development. Yoga provides a safe and structured activity that is developmentally appropriate. Yoga makes our bodies great both inside and out. It provides a means for students to find an activity that is fun and that all can participate in. It provides an important mind and body connection that seems urgent right now, as there seems to be a major disconnect in our modern society.

Our nation's public schools have an exceptional opportunity to promote healthy behaviors and reinforce the academic achievement of school-aged students. Approximately 53 million children, or 95% of children aged 5 to 17 years, attend the 117,500 elementary and secondary schools in the United States. For that reason, it is critical that health initiatives such as yoga programs in our schools and communities be a priority to help prepare students for healthy and balanced lifestyles (Burgeson et al., 2001).

WHOLE-CHILD LEARNING

Einstein once said, "We can't solve problems by using the same kind of thinking we used when we created them" (www.brainyquote.com/quotes/authors/a/albert_einstein.html). Educators, parents, schools, and communities need to foster a change—a paradigm shift. Our education system at this time tends to emphasize primarily verbal (writing) and logical (math) intelligences. The shift we must make needs to encompass educating the whole child with the intention of inclusion, individualization, and meaningful learning. Multiple intelligences or learning styles are a more-holistic approach to teaching.

Yoga and Whole-Child Learning

Yoga engages the whole student by providing activities that incorporate important intelligences or learning styles suggested by education theorists, such as visual, kinesthetic (body), musical, intuitive, and naturalist, which is the awareness of one's personal environment and interaction with nature (Gardner & Hatch, 1989; Wenig, 2003). There are two additional learning styles that yoga can significantly influence: interpersonal and intrapersonal. Interpersonal involves looking outward at the behavior, feelings, and motivation of others such as peers and parents, while intrapersonal is the individual refection of one's own feelings. Perhaps these authentic interpersonal and intrapersonal connections are what is missing from our students' lives. As a result, they turn outside of themselves to the nonreal, "virtual" connections of TV, Web sites, chat rooms, and so on. We need to provide students with inner resources such as calming, feeling centered, and self-acceptance to feel connected and whole in order to lead healthy, balanced, and fulfilling lives, which will have a positive impact on the health of the planet.

It has been estimated that students in the United States get 15 minutes or less of recess each day. According to the National Association for Sport and Physical Education, a nonprofit professional organization that sets education standards for physical education, 50% of all students and 75% of all high school students do not attend any physical education classes (www.aahperd.org/naspe/ShapeOfTheNation/template.cfm?template=pressRelease.html). Many of our students do not have opportunities for active play or after-school activities that involve physical activity. For several reasons, standards-based education reform has not embraced education of the whole child. Education reform does not provide adequate opportunities for physical activity and movement by eliminating physical education and recess in favor of more test preparation time. What this education reform does not seem to understand is that our students are kinetic learners, meaning they learn through movement, and by making students sit all day, learning is actually shut down. Our modern education offers few experiences for healthy interactive play and connection to nature. Our students have lost their natural intuition to seek out play and release stress through moving their bodies. Yoga provides experiences using all of these intelligences in ways that are fun and meaningful, and yoga has been doing this for thousands of years.

Many administrators incorrectly assume that time spent in physical activity takes away from academic achievement. This could not be further from the truth, as Carlson et al. (2008) discovered in a representative study of more than 5,000 K-5 students from all over the country. Girls who were enrolled in higher levels of physical activity (from 70 to 300 minutes per week) significantly improved their math and reading skills. No association, either positive or negative, was found between higher amounts of physical activity and standardized test scores for boys in this longitudinal study. This is an important finding for all of us who care about educating the whole child and emphasizing the importance of physical activity, including yoga.

Research to Support Yoga for our Students

A growing body of scientific research supports the benefits of yoga for adults (Raub, 2002), but there is a limited amount of research specifically on the benefits of yoga for school-aged children. A review of 15 studies involving 535 children found positive results in the social, emotional, intellectual, behavioral, and physical areas (Kassow, 2004). Unfortunately, most of the studies included in this review had numerous research design problems, making it difficult to draw definite conclusions.

There is one benchmark study that offers some promising research on the benefits of children's participation in a school-based yoga program. This 2003 study by Slovacek and colleagues investigated yoga instruction at the Accelerated School in South Central Los Angeles. Slovacek's investigation is a significant contribution to the research regarding the benefits of yoga for our students because of the nature of the school investigated, the diversity of students, and the number of students who participated. The Accelerated School, a K-8 charter school for inner-city at-risk students, is 62% Hispanic and 36% African American, and the entire school of 405 students participated in a yoga program. Participation in yoga improved student scores on flexibility, upper-body strength, and aerobic capacity. Students' academic performance in grades and in Stanford Achievement Test (SAT) scores also improved. Yoga can be an effective method of helping students improve their physical, emotional, and intellectual health as well as improving the quality of educational experiences offered in our schools.

Yoga for Stress Reduction

During the intense period of physical, emotional, social, and intellectual growth of childhood, there is a great deal of stress. When confronted with a stressor, our students have a tendency to kick into or set off the sympathetic nervous system. This is known as the familiar fight or flight response, with elevated heart rate, elevated blood pressure, and a host of other reactions that are exhausting and leave students less able to cope and with a weakened immune system, making them more vulnerable to getting sick. This stress contributes to feelings of inadequacy, low self-esteem, depression, isolation, rejection, and loss of control. The amount of stress our children face is apparent in the rising numbers of students with attention-deficit/hyperactivity disorder (ADHD); stress-related symptoms such as asthma, stomach problems, and headaches; and depression, mood disorders, and anxiety (www.extension.iastate.edu/publications/PM1660F.pdf). Violence, divorce, terrorism threats, technology, and competition are just a few of the stressors our students face, which is perhaps very different from what previous generations experienced. In addition, our students' attention is scattered in many directions—watching hundreds of television channels, gaming, surfing the Internet, text messaging—and cell phones are turned on 24-7. Multitasking is considered normal behavior. Our challenge is to provide time for students to practice mindful, proactive, healthy, and effective tools to deal with these difficult issues and distractions.

Research has shown that school curriculums that include stress-management programs improve academic performance, self-esteem, classroom conduct, concentration, and emotional balance and decrease helplessness, aggression, and behavior problems of students (Kiselica et al., 1994; Manjunath & Telles, 2004; Norlander, Moas, & Archer, 2005; Stueck & Gloeckner, 2005). Unfortunately, very few stress-management programs are being utilized in our schools. Another concern is that most of these programs may focus only on the cognitive and behavioral aspects of stress management without the more-holistic, comprehensive approach that yoga can provide, including movement, breath exercises, and relaxation.

Yoga can significantly affect our students' stress in many ways. The practice of yoga breath control is called pranayama. Pranayama encourages parasympathetic drive, also known as rest and digest, which allows the body and mind to slow down and recover, thus bringing the body and mind back into balance, or homeostasis.

Yoga can help students transfer the skill of breath control to stressful situations in school, such as taking a relaxing breath before a test. Research shows that when the breath is steady and calm, the mind and emotions can also be steady and calm.

Yoga can favorably influence our students' stress by improving self-efficacy. Self-efficacy is a student's belief in her ability to take action that will produce positive results. The greater confidence a student has in her ability to do an activity, the more likely she will stick with it and do it more often. Yoga provides a wonderful environment to foster students' motivation to keep at tasks that are difficult. This is accomplished by providing a physical challenge for growth, a means to enhance mental concentration, and activities to foster confidence. Additionally, yoga helps students cultivate an internal locus of control. This means a student takes responsibility for his own actions and experiences and does not blame what happens to him on others or things out of his control, known as external locus of control.

Yoga can also facilitate deeper and more-restful sleep for our students. Yoga emphasizes a creative outlet to balance the overly structured and stressful atmosphere of the classroom, where performance and competition dominate at the expense of imagination and spontaneous play. Yoga is a low- or no-cost quintessential stress-management program that has passed the test of time (thousands of years) because it works.

Yoga for Fighting Childhood Obesity

According to the Centers for Disease Control (CDC), the rates of obesity and inactivity among youth in the United States are staggering (www.cdc.gov/healthyyouth/overweight/index.htm). Of children aged 6 to 19, 17% are obese (more than 9 million children), and 35% of our youth do not meet the minimum requirements for regular activity. This should be a wake-up call for all those involved with the growth and development of our students to take on the challenge of keeping their bodies and minds fit for healthy and balanced living across the life span. In their busy and stressful lives, it is hard for students to be active every day with decreasing recess and physical education time; increased sitting time in school; more car and bus travel; and recreational pursuits that mostly involve sitting, such as gaming and watching media.

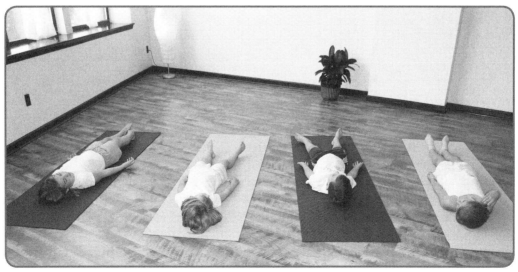

Photo Courtesy of Sara Gustavesen.

Yoga can help students learn to manage stress.

The environment that many of our students live in does not provide good messages about healthy eating, especially with food advertising and the prevalence of junk and fast food. Some students will respond to stress by overeating. Emotional eating can be a coping mechanism because eating certain foods causes the body to release dopamine, which makes you feel good. Another reason that obesity is linked to stress is that when stressed, the body releases the hormone cortisol, whose function is to store fat for emergencies. Because the body is under fight or flight, the body goes into emergency mode. Unfortunately, the fat stored by the release of cortisol is in the arteries and in the abdominal area, both serious health risks at any age. Yoga is a physical activity that encourages healthy and balanced living that could offset these overwhelming obesity rates and risks.

Yoga may be incorrectly perceived to be a passive activity that does not enhance physical fitness. However, instruction in yoga provides learning experiences in all the major focus areas of a physically educated and active person. The National Association for Sport and Physical Education (NASPE, 2004) outlines the major focus areas of a physically educated person:

- **Standard 1:** Demonstrates competency in motor skills and movement patterns needed to perform a variety of physical activities.
- **Standard 2:** Demonstrates understanding of movement concepts, principles, strategies, and tactics as they apply to the learning and performance of physical activities.
- **Standard 3:** Participates regularly in physical activity.
- **Standard 4:** Achieves and maintains a health-enhancing level of physical fitness.
- **Standard 5:** Exhibits responsible personal and social behavior that respects self and others in physical activity settings.
- **Standard 6:** Values physical activity for health, enjoyment, challenge, self-expression, and social interaction.

Reprinted from *Moving Into the Future: National Standards for Physical Education*, Second Edition with permission from the National Association for Sport and Physical Education (NASPE), 1900 Association Drive, Reston, VA 20191, USA.

Numerous school districts throughout the United States are now including yoga in their physical education curricula. The school districts of Chicago, Seattle, San Francisco, Los Angeles, and the Bronx (New York) all include yoga in their programs and provide anecdotal evidence of yoga's efficacy and importance in their curricula (Alexander, 2002; Castleman, 2002). When teaching a yoga class to a diverse group of students, it is wonderful to witness students of all shapes and sizes, physical abilities, and backgrounds all enjoying yoga together.

Yoga and Body Acceptance

Yoga may also offer a solution to the obesity epidemic by buffering the negative societal and cultural influences in regard to poor body image. Our students are continually bombarded with media-hyped scientific sound bites about the latest surgery or medication to battle obesity as well as constant negativity in our media and culture concerning body size and weight. Even with "a fix" for obesity, the roots of the problem of inadequate self-acceptance and poor self-care will still remain. Through the practice of self-awareness that yoga provides, students can shift their attention to their emotions and their own internal cues for hunger and fullness rather than external stimuli such as peers, Web sites, infomercials, and television telling them to eat, to be passive, to strive to be like others with impossible goals. Health At Every Size (HAES) is a movement which encourages accepting and respecting diverse body sizes and shapes; promoting all aspects of health including physical, emotional, spiritual, and intellectual; and promoting practices that recognize individual needs for nutrition, hunger, satiety, appetite, and pleasure. Instead of using binging, purging, starving, medications, smoking, crazy diets, and exercise regimens, all in the quest to be thin, students can use yoga as a proponent and vehicle for health at every size (www.jonrobison.net/size.html).

One participant in a teen yoga class reflected on how the lessons she experienced on the mat were also applicable "off the mat" (i.e., in her everyday life). She noticed there was a shift when she stayed with difficult emotions and feelings in her practice and did not run away. This shift allowed her to see more options when difficult emotions surfaced, when before the only option she perceived was the immediate fix of food. Yoga invites all participants to improve concentration and focus and to develop self-compassion and compassion for others; yoga provides a connection to self that no medical breakthrough ever will.

BENEFITS OF YOGA FOR SCHOOL-AGED CHILDREN

On many levels, yoga for our students can be a wonderful activity with countless benefits. You will soon see how you can best facilitate yoga for different age groups. It is important to briefly review the specific benefits for various age groups.

Yoga Benefits for Ages 4 to 6

Yoga provides an excellent activity for gross motor development and total body movement, something this age group thrives on. This age group learns through interacting with the environment physically, and yoga is a great way for them to learn this way. The emphasis is on creativity and spontaneous play. Yoga for younger children does not remotely resemble adult yoga but rather allows this group to connect with the energy and qualities of the poses rather than focusing on correctly executing poses. Yoga games are a great way to include yoga and yoga philosophy in fun and meaningful activity.

Yoga Benefits for Ages 7 to 9

Yoga can provide an opportunity for this age group to improve their gross motor skills and take on challenges in strength, agility, and endurance. This group can benefit a great deal from experiences that help them cooperate with others. Yoga provides numerous opportunities for cooperative games. For example, through problem solving, students can create new poses together. This age group can also fixate on rules or perfection. Yoga can help them let go of this preoccupation and simply enjoy activity.

Yoga Benefits for Ages 10 to 12

This group is coming into adolescence; their bodies are starting to change in enormous ways, and their connections to their peers and socialization are of incredible importance. Yoga provides a safe haven for this group to feel successful and to learn how being in a supportive atmosphere helps them grow.

These students tend to have perfectionist thinking, and they get discouraged easily when their practice is not perfect. The benefit of yoga for this group is that yoga is not competitive, something they need to be reminded of frequently. There is no ESPN for yoga—and this is a good thing! There is no competition in yoga because in yoga we take care of our own needs by exploring ways to our own personal bests and to be supported by and supportive of others—important lessons this age group needs!

Yoga Benefits for Teens

Yoga is fast gaining popularity among teens, as it can provide both a physical outlet and a challenge. While traditional sports or recreation may turn teens off because of competition, rules, cost, lack of access, or focus on athletic ability, yoga can provide a meaningful and enjoyable physical workout. The teenage years tend to be a time of disconnect for teens from the vast changes their bodies are going through as they mature. Yoga is easy to learn, fun, and safe, and it provides a nurturing and inclusive atmosphere. Yoga provides a way for teens to find balance when they are at odds with their schoolwork, families, friends, bodies, and raging hormones.

During the teen years, students start to define their own identities and explore possible paths and choices in the midst of the expectations that society, their peers, and their parents have of them. Yoga for teens allows for self-study and self-care as well as development of vital intrapersonal and interpersonal intelligence skills such as improved communication skills, which are critically needed at this developmental stage.

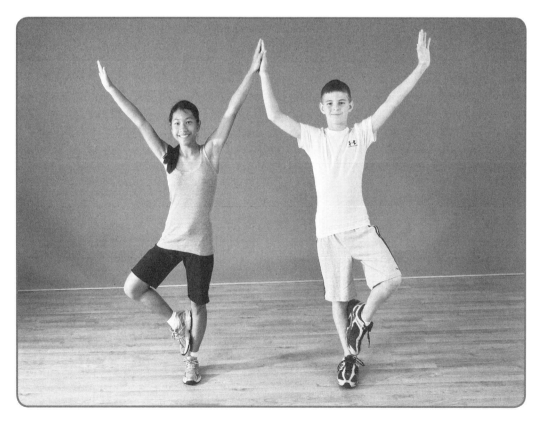

Yoga gives students the opportunity to socialize in a supportive environment.

Yoga Benefits for Student-Athletes

The benefits of yoga for student-athletes include increasing their cardiorespiratory fitness, strength, flexibility, and overall fitness. Yoga emphasizes a balanced athlete. Many student-athletes have a limited range of motion, muscles with limited strength and imbalances, poor cardiorespiratory endurance, or excess body fat. Some athletes are more dominant and strong on the right side of their bodies or abdominally strong but with weak or inflexible lower backs. For example, a soccer player may have limited upper-body strength. Being unbalanced makes an athlete prone to injury. The poses in yoga, particularly the standing and balancing poses, require sustained isometric contraction and balanced muscular effort. The continued movement in yoga can allow for sufficient heart rate response for cardiorespiratory training of low to moderate intensity. Yoga postures improve the body's alignment, resulting in increased circulation, nervous system stimulation, and increased energy (Bauman, 2002).

However, just as it is important to educate the whole child, it is equally important to develop the whole athlete. In sports training, there is a tendency to train and emphasize only specific and narrow aspects of fitness such as power and intensity, with a result of becoming rigid and unbalanced in both mind and body. Although training physically is what most athletes feel they need to do to be better and win, the crux of training is really in the mind domain. For example, many of our student-athletes train to perform mechanically or automatically without mindfulness of muscle stretch or action. This imbalance encourages dropout, injury, and detachment from the body, ignoring an inner wisdom about what is best for one's health. Damaging axioms such as "no pain, no gain" encourage athletes not to listen to their bodies. Without the concentration, focus, introspection, and paying attention to sensation, proper alignment, and body mechanics that yoga can provide, youth can injure themselves or become unmotivated because of staleness or lack of improvement (e.g., they just go through the motions).

A disconnection is often seen in student-athletes, such as burnout. They may state, "It just isn't fun anymore" because of all the pressure to win and perform. The importance of the term *student-athlete* needs to be emphasized, with a priority on learning, academics, and balance. Today, student-athletes find themselves juggling many different responsibilities. They must have enough mental strength and stamina to study, work hard as an athlete, and enjoy a social life. Yoga can offer a change of perspective to allow an athlete to look not just at the physical aspects of training but also to recognize the spirituality behind yoga, which is the desire to meet one's best potential and do things in life "for the love of it." For example, through yoga a student-athlete can focus on "What are you bringing to this team? What are your strengths?" These questions are focused on gaining a positive mental attitude about oneself and not what others expect. Everything envisioned in yoga is positive; failure, problems, and excuses are put aside. The student practices being present during yoga sessions, and this skill could transfer to competing or studying, where a distraction detracts from putting forth one's best effort.

Other yoga practices such as mental imagery allow players to picture in their minds what they are trying to do. For example, athletes could imagine themselves pitching the perfect pitch. They can "practice" in their minds, and this will positively influence their ability to perform in real situations. If during a game or practice session things get rocky, players have practiced over and over again in yoga to take a deep breath, to take a moment to center and become grounded. Yoga sessions with athletes can be supplemented by activities such as setting intentions by repeating positive self-statements (called affirmations) or setting goals with the use of a training diary to record both physical and mental factors. Athletes can seek inspiration by reading biographies of motivating athletes and also volunteer to mentor younger athletes, thus embracing the whole yogic athlete.

Yoga Benefits for Students With Special Needs

Yoga has been shown to be an effective stress-management tool, particularly for students with learning or behavioral challenges. For students with attention-deficit/ hyperactivity disorder (ADHD), yoga improved on-task time and attention and reduced symptoms in primary grade ADHD children (Peck et al., 2005) and boys in treatment for ADHD (Jensen & Kenny, 2004).

Yoga has been used to help at-risk youth around the United States, and it is seen as an important outlet for students who have behavioral problems, have spent time in the juvenile justice system, or have failed at traditional school settings. Programs such as the Lineage Project (www.lineageproject.org) based in New York and the West Hollywood Opportunity School, a Los Angeles alternative public high school, provide meditation, yoga, and awareness-based practices for at-risk and incarcerated youth (Stukin, 2001). Yoga is offered as a structured, age-appropriate activity to help teenage prostitutes deal with stress at the Children of the Night residential program in Van Nuys, California (www.childrenofthenight.org/program. html). Street Yoga provides free yoga and wellness education to youth living on the streets, girls in foster care, children of homeless families, and young people recovering from abuse and trauma in the Pacific Northwest (www.streetyoga.org). The mission of the Art of Yoga Project is to use yoga and self-expression (through writing, painting, and photographs) as tools for well-being and empowerment for at-risk adolescent girls (www.theartofyogaproject.org/background.php). These are just a few examples of grassroots organizations whose missions are grounded in the belief in the numerous benefits of yoga for all children.

Yoga has also been shown to be an effective teaching tool when working with students with Down syndrome, cerebral palsy, autism, sensory integration disorder, and learning difficulties (Klimas, 2003; Sumar, 1998). The ability of a special needs student to focus, attend, and follow directions in fine and gross motor activities can be improved through yoga. The emphasis of yoga is and has always been inclusion of participants of all abilities. For example, yoga can be easily adapted to students in wheelchairs or with other developmental challenges. Teaching with the intention of inclusion and adapting for the success of all are natural elements of yoga.

SUMMARY

Our students are faced with enormous challenges and stressors in accelerated, negatively charged, and disconnected environments that do not encourage optimal learning. Yoga can offer an inexpensive and simple integrative learning tool where students are allowed to enjoy being challenged and feel good about meeting those challenges without comparing themselves with others. Yoga helps our students feel better about themselves and address whole-child learning. Yoga has been found to be a wonderful physical activity for all ages and allows students to experience stress reduction, body acceptance, and improved academic performance. Yoga can also be of benefit to student-athletes and students with special needs. The next chapters will guide you in bringing the gifts of yoga to your students!

chapter

2

Yoga for Healthy, Balanced Living

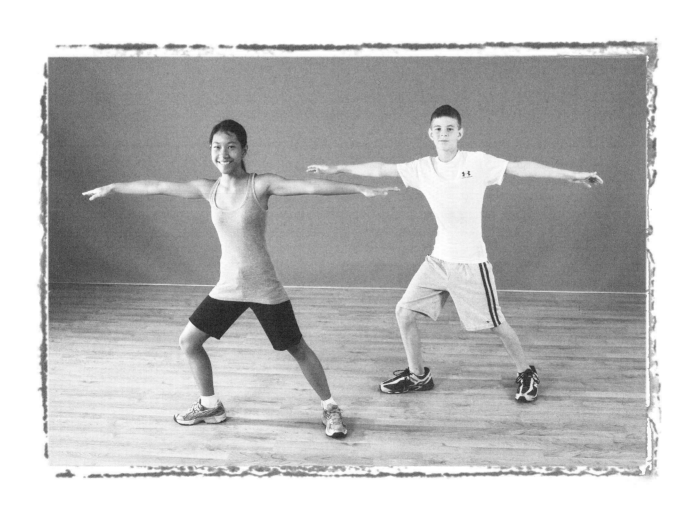

Yoga provides experiences to develop healthy and balanced living through physical postures, breathing, and relaxation and also includes strategies to live a balanced and healthy life. This chapter discusses yoga's philosophy and guidelines that allow students to learn valuable tools in class that can be transferred to everyday life. These tools include managing stress and encouraging well-being; providing focus and concentration; and becoming more mindful, confident, responsible, introspective, reflective, and self-directed. Yoga also allows students to cultivate better relationships with themselves, better relationships with others, and a oneness with a higher purpose. The skills that yoga helps build include tolerance and compassion for imperfection, inadequacies, differences, and challenges—in both ourselves and others.

DEFINING YOGA

The English translation of the word *yoga* is yoke. A yoke is used to join things together, and in yoga this means to connect the body, spirit, and mind holistically (meaning "to the whole"). The numerous benefits of yoga highlighted in the first chapter, which cover the scope of improved physical fitness and feeling more emotionally healthy and mentally focused, are due to this holistic approach. When we focus on only one part of physical fitness, such as muscle strength, the body is unbalanced and can become vulnerable to injury. Similarly, when we separate the mind and spirit from the body, we are left unbalanced, disconnected, and not whole. In yoga, the goal is to strengthen and stretch our bodies in order to quiet and slow down our racing minds and to cultivate an inner stillness and awareness.

Yoga is not a religion but a philosophy and set of guidelines—not rules—that assist in making better decisions and creating a better quality of life. These principles are not based on any religion, dogma, or belief system and do not contradict but rather complement any belief system or faith. Although yoga originates from ancient India, it is not a form of Hinduism or any religion. Yoga is a holistic practice that brings together the spirit, mind, and body, allowing each person to decide how her practice best meets her needs. The intention of yoga is the approach of taking what you need from yoga and putting the rest back with respect. People will utilize different aspects of yoga at different times in their lives, and hence it is a practice that can be used through the life span. Yoga has enough flexibility to honor this individualized approach, so no one is left out or alienated.

Yoga is referred to as a practice, meaning a process to be worked on over and over again for a lifetime. There is no destination or final outcome. On the other hand, exercise might be seen as a task or a goal that we might perform during a certain time in our lives such as playing for a high school sports team. Once it is over, participants stop being active.

A tree is often used to symbolize the many aspects or branches of yoga. All of us can relate to the beauty of trees: the foundation of deep roots; the strength of the trunk; the movement of the branches, twigs, and leaves. The trunk of the tree represents the different goals of yoga:

- Raja yoga focuses on the ultimate purpose of yoga: to practice meditation.
- Karma yoga is where we practice yoga in order to serve others and make the world a better place.
- Jnana yoga is where we explore the intellect of the heart.

The yoga we offer to our students for healthy and balanced living incorporates all these types of yoga. Within the branches of yoga, we can go into more depth regarding the guidelines for meaningful and purposeful life. We explore these guidelines or suggestions in yoga, yet the breadth and depth of the exploration is up to the individual.

EIGHT BRANCHES FOR A MEANINGFUL, PURPOSEFUL LIFE

Often yoga is seen as a physical practice with an emphasis on suppleness and agility. Some people think yoga is not for them, especially if they are flexibility challenged. However, yoga's roots are deeply embedded in "yoking," meaning to join together the individual self with the true self to answer the questions "Who am I?" and "Why am I here?" The basic yoga teachings were gathered and organized about 200 BC by the sage Patanjali. These texts, known as the Yoga Sutras, still guide yoga today and are organized into eight practical branches or paths (see figure 2.1).

The timeless and universal framework that yoga provides is a model for all aspects of healthy and balanced living. The eight branches of yoga for healthy and balanced living include the following:

- **Yamas** are ethical guidelines for relationships.
- **Niyamas** are positive habits or behaviors.
- **Asanas** are the physical yoga poses or postures.
- **Pranayamas** are the focused breathing exercises.
- **Pratyahara** means turning inward of the senses.
- **Dharana** means concentration and the ability to focus.
- **Dhyana** means meditation practices.
- **Samadhi** is the culminating experience of connection.

This section goes into each of these important branches, explaining why these are timeless lessons our students need in order to live healthy and balanced lives.

All the branches of yoga influence each other, as do all the tenets of wellness—they are all interconnected (see figure 2.2). Students realize that making themselves calmer influences their learning, their social interactions, and their physical state—none of these are separate but an integrated whole.

Wellness is also seen as a lifelong process (see figure 2.3). It is important that yoga instructors and students recognize the value and honor of all aspects of the eight branches, or paths. The physical aspects of the asanas and breathing may act as an important stepping-stone that might allow participants to appreciate and embrace the mental and spiritual paths as well. We can help students appreciate yoga's ancient philosophy in modern times in ways that are meaningful, healthy, and rewarding.

Branch One: Yamas

The first branch of yoga is known as yamas, which are considered the ethical guidelines for healthy relationships. The relationships emphasized here are not only with others but also with ourselves—the most important relationship of all. The five yamas, or guidelines, are known as Ahimsa, Satya, Asteya, Brahmacharya, and Aparigraha.

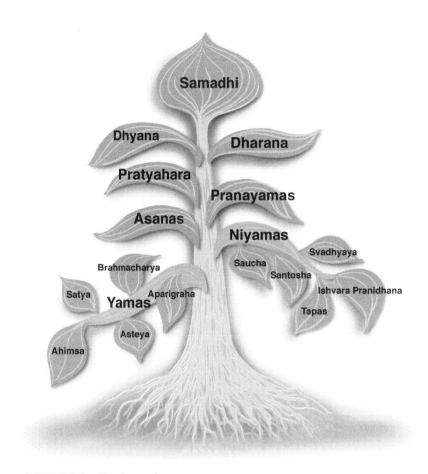

FIGURE 2.1   The tree of yoga.

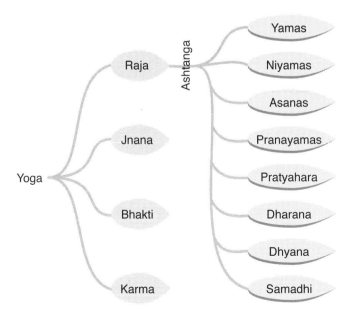

FIGURE 2.2   The eight branches of yoga.

Ahimsa

The first yama guideline is Ahimsa, which means nonharming and nonviolence and is the foundation from which all yoga must grow. It is easy to relate to Ahimsa, which translates to what is known as the golden rule: "Do unto others, as you would want done unto you." Ahimsa guides us toward compassion for both self and others by being kind and treating others as we want to be treated. Practicing yoga with the intention of nonharming allows students to stay alert and become self-reliant and nonjudgmental, without any shame about their bodies, emotions, and

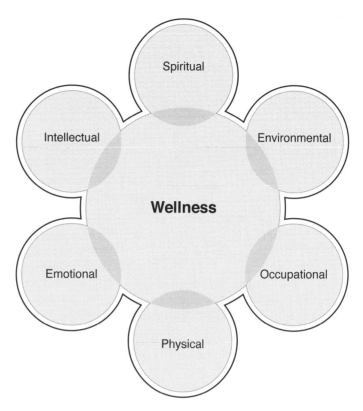

FIGURE 2.3 The wellness wheel.

feelings. This promotes self-acceptance and deepens the relationship with oneself. Ahimsa also promotes the concept of self-care. In this technological age, students need to critically evaluate a copious amount of health information, products, and services. Self-care is when people make decisions based on what is best for them and are not persuaded by peers or fancy advertising.

Satya

The second yama is Satya, which means to have an attitude of being truthful and honest in our words, thoughts, and actions. Students learn to practice Satya when they value being truthful to themselves as well as avoid situations where they might have to deviate from their truth. We can encourage students to use language that is assertive of their own beliefs and to use their voices when situations become out of hand or risky. Students also learn to cultivate critical radar for information and messages that are not true and honest. For example, students would apply critical thinking to information they may get from the Internet by making sure to check for valid and reliable resources and not simply accepting that if it is printed online, it must be true.

Asteya

The third yama is Asteya, which translates as "nonstealing" and means to not take things that do not belong to you. This would mean for our students to respect others' privacy and possessions, to not take advantage of someone's generosity, and to not take credit for something they did not do. Asteya means developing a personal style and just being ourselves instead of copying someone else's style. This requires being creative and honoring our own ideas.

Brahmacharya

Brahmacharya, the fourth yama, cultivates the attitude of self-control. This yama encourages practicing moderation (e.g., not overeating or watching too much television). Moderation is an important concept for our students, as they are constantly bombarded with messages such as "More is better" or "Supersize!" In yoga, the taking of the middle path, or moderation, means trying a challenging yoga pose with enough effort to explore and take it into more depth but at the same time finding ease and acceptance. The story *Goldilocks and the Three Bears* comes to mind with Brahmacharya—"not too much, not too little, but what feels just right." Brahmacharya also promotes an important concept of delayed gratification. Many of the important goals in our lives take time and discipline, and in turn they become more satisfying and lasting.

Aparigraha

The final yama is Aparigraha, which means not being greedy, taking only what you really need. George Shaw once said, "There are two tragedies in life. One is to lose your heart's desire. The other is to gain it" (www.brainyquote.com/quotes/quotes/g/georgebern161559.html). We are culturally ingrained to want and addicted to consuming and acquiring more and more: "I need to have this newest video game" or "I have to buy a pair of high-tech sneakers." Aparigraha encourages simplification instead of accumulating and hoarding more stuff. This could be integrated into the classroom by encouraging reusing, recycling, and renewing. Another example of a way to include the guideline of Aparigraha is to have the students research unnecessary deforestation and excessive use of natural resources. They could then become advocates for using products that do not encourage deforestation, using fewer natural resources, and making the campus more environmentally friendly, or green.

Branch Two: Niyamas

The second branch of yoga, consisting of the principles called the niyamas, involves developing positive habits or behaviors important for healthy and balanced living. These principles allow people to act in a way that is harmonious with what is of value to them. The five niyamas include Saucha, Santosha, Tapas, Svadhyaya, and Ishvara Pranidhana.

Saucha

The first niyama is Saucha and is the habit of cleanliness and purity. On the physical health level, we teach good hygiene to our students. Students also learn about nutritious foods that keep the body running clean and the mind fueled. At school, Saucha can be cultivated by keeping the environment clean—our school, classroom, work areas, and even our rooms at home—by keeping things tidy and organized and not letting clutter take over our spaces. By taking the concept of cleanliness to a more-holistic point of view, we also teach "being clean" in our thinking and speaking. Students can be encouraged to develop positive thoughts and affirmations and to speak respectfully without curse words. We can ask students to clean up their language, noting that words of putting each other down won't be tolerated in yoga.

Santosha

Santosha is the habit of contentment, optimism, and gratitude. When a student practices mindfulness, she stays present in the moment and focused on what she is doing and feeling right now without worrying about the past or future. Santosha helps students develop the habit of getting "unstuck" from times when they might feel sorry for themselves or frustrated when something is not working out. It brings the focus back to right now, to figuring out what they can proactively do about the situation or their reaction to the situation. The concept of locus of control is the perception of our ability to be responsible for the outcomes of our actions. Santosha allows students to accept situations and people as they are and to let go of the struggle to change or manipulate what they cannot change. Santosha suggests that students view challenges as opportunities. Santosha cultivates the habit in students of taking responsibility for their own experience by asking them to look at their yoga practice as a source of optimism, contentment, and gratitude.

Tapas

Tapas is the habit of self-discipline, the determination to keep goals, do our best, and use our energy to do positive things. This habit promotes self-efficacy. Self-efficacy is the belief in our ability to accomplish a goal or change a behavior. Tapas is the central theme in the story *The Little Engine That Could*, when the engine keeps repeating "I think I can, I think I can" as it chugs up the mountain. When a student increases his self-efficacy, he changes the way he perceives challenges. His vocabulary changes from "I wish I can" or "Maybe I can" to "I can do this!"

Svadhyaya

Svadhyaya is the habit of self-study, to be introspective, learn from mistakes, and make things better the next time a challenging situation presents itself. Svadhyaya cultivates self-awareness and reflection on "Who am I?" by asking students to notice recurring ineffective patterns and taking steps to change these patterns. A student may notice she is disappointed with the grade she received on her science fair project. Through some reflection, she might consider the amount of time and planning and see the need to work on the project regularly next time instead of leaving it to the last minute.

Ishvara Pranidhana

The final niyama healthy habit is called Ishvara Pranidhana. This is the habit of looking for meaning in the world, of answering the question "Why am I here?" We are all an important part of this universe. This habit encourages us to build trust in our intuition and to look beyond the black and white of what is in front of us to the wonders and miracles in this world. Just as we ask students to approach each yoga pose with openness, we can also ask students to open their minds to all possibilities of finding their own special contribution to the world. The attitudes and habits of the yamas and niyamas are practiced over and over in yoga, so there can be a transfer of learning to other life habits that are always self-honoring and respectful of others.

Branch Three: Asanas

The third branch of yoga is the physical practice of postures, or asanas. They are the workout of yoga. In the Eastern concept of disease, when energy (or prana) becomes stagnant, restricted, or blocked, the body is more susceptible to physiological disease or dysfunction. And the mind is more prone to psychological disease or disorders. For example, when the body is inactive from sitting all day or we hold tension in muscles or organs (e.g., backaches, headaches, or indigestion), we become stressed, anxious, and unable to perform necessary tasks. Yoga poses allow for a process of realignment of the physical body structure so that energy can circulate freely through the body.

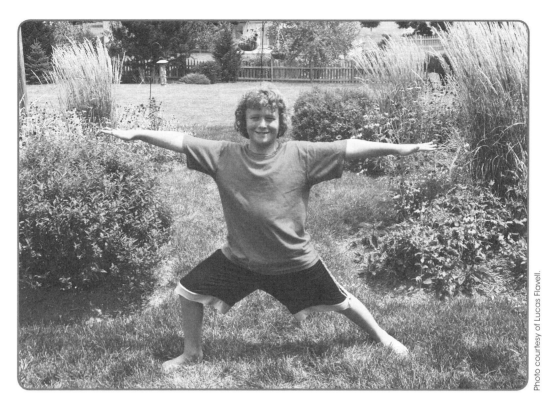

Photo courtesy of Lucas Flavell.

Asanas, or postures, make up the third branch of yoga.

The sage of yoga, Patanjali, offers the interpretation of asana as being steady and comfortable in the midst of a challenge. When we explore yoga poses, we encourage growth by challenging ourselves but without pain. This is referred to in yoga as finding "the edge." The edge is the line between stimulating growth by holding a muscle or muscle group in a strength pose or holding a stretch in a way that is calm, grounded, and breath centered. By constantly paying attention and finding "the edge," students can learn that they can stay calm and centered in the middle of a challenge when things get difficult rather than fight it or give up.

Hatha yoga is often the generic name for the physical aspects of yoga, but it has more depth and refers to the union of opposites: the sun and moon. Sun poses are postures or movements that encourage heat, openness, and outward movement. Sun poses are always balanced with moon poses, which embody cooling, healing, and receptiveness. Students learn the importance of the balance of opposites in yoga. For example, while learning a sport skill, students may emphasize only the aspects of strength or speed. But in yoga, there is an exploration of the contrasting aspects such as effort and letting go, hard and soft, courage and contentment, solid and flowing. By learning various asanas, students can choose specific yoga poses to provide their needs for nurturing, healing, energy, balance, or equanimity. This is instead of perhaps trying to meet their needs through food, caffeine, or other distractions when feeling tired, anxious, or upset. For example, forward bends help soothe the nervous system, while back bends encourage awakening.

Branch Four: Pranayamas

The fourth branch, pranayamas, means breath awareness. Breath can be thought of as the link between the mind and body and is the symbol of life. The breath is the tool to help us feel grounded, centered, and calm in the present moment, as it is never in the past or in the future. Breath awareness provides instant feedback on what is best in every moment. The breath is also the real teacher in yoga by signaling us when we have pushed too far; the breath gets caught, stuck, anxious, or scattered. Yoga without focusing on breath is like skiing without snow—you are just going through the motions! Remember that yoga means to yoke, to bring together the body, mind, and spirit, and pranayamas give us the bridge. It allows us to move from the outward, active practice of the physical poses, or asanas, and connect to the internal, stepping-inward practice that leads to calming the mind, keeping focused, and being present and mindful. When awareness of breath is linked with attention to the body, there is harmony and synchronicity. This interconnectedness cultivates confidence, strength, and flexibility on many levels, not just at the physical level. Chapter 6 offers a wide variety of breath exercises to introduce to your students.

Branch Five: Pratyahara

The fifth branch is pratyahara and translates to "withdrawal of senses." In yoga this means learning how to become aware of our senses by turning inward and turning off constant external distractions while at the same time letting go or detaching from our attitudes and judgments. An example is feeling the sensation of a tight hamstring and bringing your awareness and breath to this body region without reacting to thoughts such as "I can't touch my toes" or "Look at that kid next to me putting his palms on the floor." The key to pratyahara is awakening to the fact that thoughts take us away from our present experience. The goal of pratyahara is not to tune out but rather to tune in: to find a nice, quiet place of stillness and calm inside and not get caught up in the chaos when things get too fast, too much, and too loud.

Branches Six and Seven: Dharana and Dhyana

The two branches of dharana and dhyana are included together because they bring together two important concepts in yoga. Dharana means to develop concentration, and dhyana is meditation.

Dharana

Dharana, the sixth branch, is the cultivation of concentration and being fully present. This means not detaching and entertaining the mind while the body physically works. The Western model of fitness might encourage watching a television program or movie while walking on a treadmill, or taking a "boot camp fitness class" where the instructor yells and berates us to work harder. The goal in yoga is to develop the concentration and patience to stay awake, focused, and present in the body and mind—to really "show up" and not just go through the motions. Students need to be responsible for their own experience, to be self-directed learners, to challenge themselves in all styles of learning, and to not be afraid if things do not come easily and shy away from experiences that could be beneficial and fun. The focus on breath is an important tool to help concentrate and stay anchored in the present, as it is difficult to think about the past or dive into the future when the awareness and focus is on the breath.

Dhyana

Dhyana is the seventh branch, which encourages practicing meditation. Often meditation evokes images of painfully sitting cross-legged in some hypnotic altered state. Meditation is when our scattered "monkey-brain thoughts," those thoughts that swing wildly from branch to branch, can become quiet and instead we can

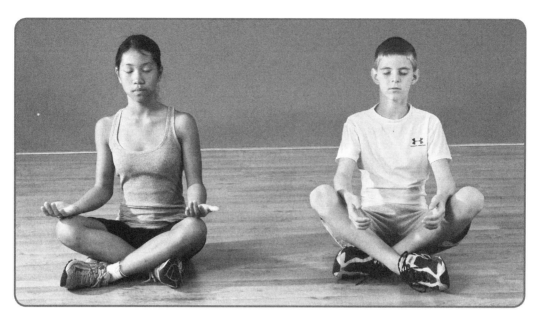

Dhyana the seventh branch, encourages meditation to quiet the mind.

concentrate or reflect on one thing. Meditation does not need to take place while seated but can be done in the simple act of walking. Students can walk quietly and softly without touching anyone and pay attention solely (bad pun) to the feeling of the foot making contact with the ground. Students could go outside for a meditation walk and reflect on all the colors of green they see and nothing else. When they get distracted (and they will), try to gently cue them to come back to the feeling of their feet on the ground or looking for the color green.

The breath can easily be used as a meditation tool as well. Asking students to pick a particular aspect of the breath, such as when their bellies rise on the inhale, can help students bring their focus inward and become meditative. The benefit of meditation is helping students quiet down enough to be able to listen to their inner voices and become reflective and responsible human beings.

Branch Eight: Samadhi

Samadhi is the final branch and refers to connection to the universe in an awakened body and mind, to feeling completely whole and well. Making the connection that our individual actions and thoughts have an impact on the rest of the world is a powerful lesson from yoga. Since yoga means to yoke, our students learn to connect with nature, the world, and taking care of the planet through their experiences learned in yoga class. Our students learn we are not separate, isolated, or lonely but an important part of this world. The final branch of samadhi is self-actualization, which means realizing our fullest potential and purpose on this earth. Einstein provides an eloquent quote that summarizes samadhi well:

A human being is a part of a whole, called by us "universe," a part limited in time and space. He experiences himself, his thoughts and feelings as something separated from the rest . . . a kind of optical delusion of his consciousness. This delusion is a kind of prison for us, restricting us to our personal desires and to affection for a few persons nearest to us. Our task must be to free ourselves from this prison by widening our circle of compassion to embrace all living creatures and the whole of nature in its beauty. (www.quotationspage.com/quote/5073.html)

SUMMARY

Yoga provides experiential activities to allow our students to explore all of these eight branches. The wellness model of holistic health suggests the balance, integration, and harmony of physical, emotional, intellectual, spiritual, social, and environmental components of health. The eight branches of yoga closely parallel and complement this model.

Yoga at first glance may appear to be yet another physical fitness craze on America's trendy radar. What is remarkable about sharing yoga with our students is its depth and breadth. This may seem overwhelming to beginners, but keep in mind that it is a lifelong practice and study. One doesn't become a yoga master or expert but studies and practices yoga throughout the life span. Yoga's gift will unfold itself to you and your students time and time again. The eight branches of yoga are the tools for healthy and balanced living. Within the scope of yoga for our school-aged students, the philosophical principles offered here are a foundation. There are numerous other principles in yoga, and the guidelines included here are not all-encompassing but are presented as simply as possible and in ways that can be meaningful and empowering for both you and your students. Instructors are encouraged to further explore the vast depth and breadth of the learning yoga can offer. Please see the reference section for additional resources on yoga philosophy.

The next chapter helps us create a yoga learning environment that will embrace the wonderful tree of yoga.

chapter

3

Teaching Effective Yoga Classes

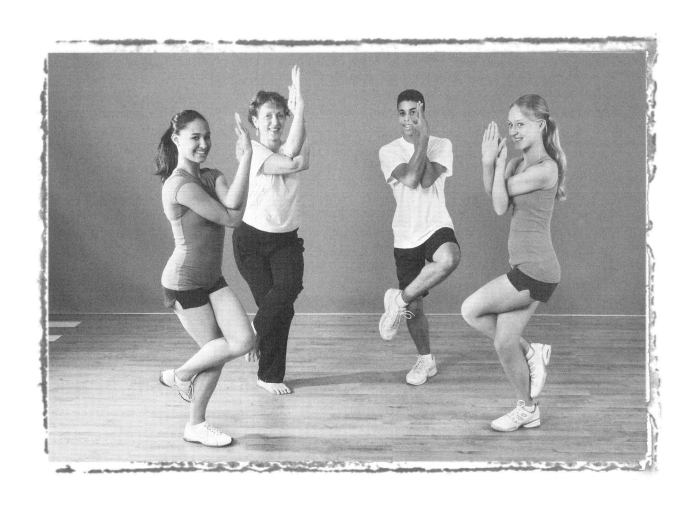

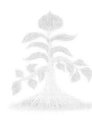

*P*arker Palmer states the following in his book *The Courage to Teach: Exploring the Inner Landscape of a Teacher's Life*: "Many of us became teachers for reasons of the heart, animated by a passion for some subject and for helping people learn. . . . But many of us lose heart as the years of teaching go by. How can we take heart in teaching once more so that we can, as good teachers always do, give heart to our students?" (p. 17). This quote struck me as the reason I started teaching yoga. I had taught human movement for many years, and the gift of yoga came along at a time when I thought I had lost my heart for teaching.

An effective yoga class provides a positive learning environment, which includes a motivating climate for both the teacher and the students; a creative, safe, and nurturing learning experience; and meaningful instruction and feedback. This chapter provides strategies to teach effective and enjoyable yoga to your students.

The chapter discusses the important qualities of a yoga instructor working with children. It introduces methods to create motivating classes through class structure, classroom management, and teaching strategies that help students learn. In addition, strategies for creative learning experiences for specific age groups are reviewed.

COMPONENTS OF THE YOGA CLASS

A yoga class includes the dynamics of the yoga teacher and the students in a climate that is individualized and rooted in an atmosphere of self-responsibility. This asks the teacher to allow students to take responsibility for their own experience and safety through instruction that embraces and respects the whole child. Yoga creates a climate where students are encouraged to focus inward and pay attention to their own experiences rather than expect the teacher to do this for them. Teaching yoga requires the teacher, the students, and the environment to embrace a dynamic that is motivating, safe, and respectful for all.

The Yoga Teacher

Whether the instructor has taught adult yoga or group exercise classes or has taught children but never yoga, it is important that the instructor keep the intention of being open and making yoga fun and playful—in yoga we do this in all classes no matter what the age. As an instructor, you do not want to be an entertainer; rather, you want to create an atmosphere that encourages participants to explore and enjoy creating their own experiences.

A great deal of traditional physical education eliminates participants and forces students to compete, to follow restrictive rules, and to sit and wait while others get their turns. Yoga for healthy and balanced living is the opposite. In the late 1970s and early 1980s, several philosophical movements emerged within physical education such as movement exploration and New Games. The emphasis of these movements was creative exploration and learning through human movement that was student centered. An example of using a movement exploration approach is teaching the skill of bouncing a ball and asking the students to discover how many ways they can bounce a ball without using their hands. In the movement called New Games, the mantra is no rules, everyone plays, and no one gets hurt. The noise and energy level using this explorative approach can be high, but there is also a great deal of creativity and fun happening! This is exactly what yoga for our students should be. Yoga has embraced the philosophies of these movements and has stood the test of time as the oldest distinct practice for self-development. We engage the students in creative ways that allow them to enjoy movement, use their imaginations, control their impulses, and learn to relax.

A passion for teaching is what is most important when working with students. When the instructor is enthusiastic and passionate, it is hard for students not to catch on to this energy. Teaching is a relationship between the teacher and the student. In yoga, this relationship is about facilitation for a great deal of the time. Providing facilitation means helping students explore and find the answers for themselves rather than instructing where the students might copy or mimic the teacher. This can be accomplished in both the instructor and the student by cultivating a beginner's mind. Having a beginner's mind means approaching each and every yoga session as an opportunity to learn something new and have fun. This also reduces expectations that the teacher is the expert or a guru and shows that the instructor is just a fellow yogi—meaning a student of yoga. The bottom line is, if the instructor has as her foundation a love of teaching, then yoga can and will become part of that love, and it becomes very gratifying to share the gift of yoga.

Factors to Engage Students in Yoga

Bringing a passion for learning is important for any instructor. It is also crucial to keep in mind some of the psychological factors necessary for participation to help spark a student's interest. The first factor is self-efficacy, which is a person's belief in his ability to perform a task. As discussed in the benefits of yoga, yoga helps improve a student's self-efficacy by the inherent nature of an activity that is not competitive and without judgment. Success breeds success, and self-efficacy can be realized through authentic and meaningful experience and feedback. Internal locus of control is another factor in participation. This means the student perceives that she is in control, and her experience and subsequent success are not dependent on others such as her coach or parent. Intrinsic motivation means participation in an activity for the sheer pleasure and satisfaction of participation and not for an external reward such as a trophy or promotion to a higher rank or a harder league. One way we can help students realize intrinsic motivation is drawing their attention to the positive feelings of participation. Finally, a positive social support is important. Setting a climate of respect and inclusion in each class will foster positive social support.

Creating a Motivating Yoga Environment

As a yoga instructor, you are a powerful force in developing loving and caring students. This begins by modeling the same attributes students need to learn of remaining gentle, being noncompetitive, and being nonjudgmental. This can be encouraged by creating classes that are student centered and cooperative, by honoring the experience and contributions of all, and by helping students choose responsible behavior. To create this motivating climate for learning, make sure to greet each student by name. Make the time to learn about your students' interests and dreams. Feel free to share your personality, stories, sense of humor, silly jokes, and laughter—this is part of the joy of teaching. In addition, encourage students to share their stories and jokes in class.

A critical aspect of establishing a motivating climate is to have students own the class experience. This means that students, no matter what their age, share in the responsibility of establishing a positive climate for the class. Yoga can provide a unique opportunity for students to be involved in the learning process. Asking students for their input, having them be involved in planning, and providing them with options in their tasks are all ways to allow students to share in the ownership of the learning process. Younger students may share in chores such as setting up the room or putting things away. Older students could assist in teaching the class or be in charge of the music or a specific aspect of class, such as a poem they would share during the final relaxation.

Creating Positive Student and Teacher Energy

The yoga experience should tell students that what they have to say and contribute is important and valued. This might mean stepping back from always having an answer or comment and accepting what is being said by the students without judgment or emphasizing that they are not alone with the feelings they may be experiencing, such as anxiety or frustration. A significant aspect of listening is to listen with the eyes by noticing the students' body language. For example, a student feeling anxious and unable to settle down in class needs calm acceptance and assurance by the instructor.

Preparation is a significant task in teaching, and often as teachers, we put a great deal of time and effort into our lesson plans. Yoga challenges us not only to prepare the best we can as good educators but also to pay attention to students' energy. Often in a yoga class, you will notice students spontaneously finding ways to balance their energy. For example, after a vigorous pose, students find a restorative pose to help them rest and restore themselves. This is an important skill to help students find the right balance in their energy. When the group seems very tired, a class with more restorative poses might be in order, or stopping the more-active poses early and extending the relaxation phase might be best.

Yoga can be a fantastic tool when students' energy and attention become distracted, and subsequently the students become frustrated. "Monkey brain" occurs when one's thoughts swing like a monkey from branch to branch, and it may be hard to practice a challenging pose. Help a student slow down these racing thoughts, calm down, and feel less scattered by encouraging the student to become focused on the breath and to keep calm and still while holding a pose. Use a helpful cue such as "Can you freeze your pose but keep your breath strong?" Students can also be cued to perform a body check: systematically checking or scanning the body, noticing tension in any specific body part, and then relaxing the body part. In chapter 6, there are several exercises for students to use their imagination to help them connect to and relax their bodies.

Creating Respect for Self, Class, and Others

In establishing a caring learning community, students need to be respectful of themselves and others. There are several concepts to keep in mind in cultivating this respect. One of these concepts is, there are no perfect poses; the students need to be encouraged to steer away from competition and judgment of themselves or the poses. Instead, encourage the students to move intuitively with awareness while paying attention to what feels right to them.

An example of this is introducing the turtle pose. In this pose, the students sit on the floor, with their legs extended straight out and separated about 2 feet (.6 meters) apart in the shape of a V (see figure 3.1). The students then hinge at the hips and reach forward, taking hold of the feet, ankles, or lower legs. This is not an easy pose and takes the sincere intention of slow progress and patience.

It is natural to gravitate or play favorites toward certain poses that come easy and to dislike the poses that are challenging. Yoga asks us to not label poses as good or bad but to take what we need from all of them to help us grow. The task is not performing the poses the right way but allowing the students to find what

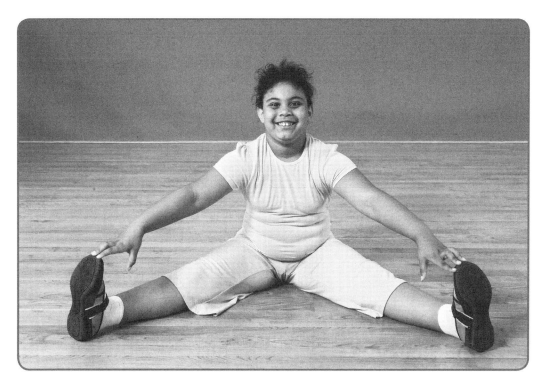

FIGURE 3.1 Turtle pose.

they can learn from each pose or to emulate the meaning or intention of each pose. However, do watch to make sure that students are doing poses safely. Even though yoga does not aim for the "best" pose, it is still important to do poses in a way that won't harm the students.

What is so beautiful about the yoga poses is they metaphorically capture ancient virtues. In the case of the turtle, the lesson is tenacity and determination and not necessarily taking the fast track or looking for the quick fix to solve a problem. While practicing the turtle as just described, the students can think about perhaps a goal they have that requires some of these same virtues the turtle emulates and set their intention toward accomplishing this goal. Yoga provides the practice for students to develop skills that go beyond the classroom. In the case of the turtle pose, the lesson learned is not everything is going to come easy, and most of the time we learn the most from the harder challenges. Among the numerous skills garnered from yoga that transfer to the classroom are patience, calming, focus, problem solving, creativity, self-confidence, and the energy to face challenges in a proactive way.

In cultivating respect in yoga, ownership is a concept that ties in here as well. Ownership means taking responsibility for your own experience and paying attention to what is best for yourself. Instructors can use what is called permission language— statements that cue the students to continuously give themselves permission to do what is best for them. Permission language asks students to find creative ways to modify a pose to find a simpler variation without feeling they are not doing enough or what everyone else might be doing. An example of permission language is "If it feels right for you, try finding a way to stretch deeper into this pose."

Part of the ownership of practicing yoga is honoring individual needs in a respectful way. It is critical that students not distract from others' experience by becoming a distraction when discouraged. For example, if a student needs to stop holding a yoga pose before the rest of the class, which is called "coming out of the pose," she should not distract the rest of the class by making unnecessary noise or comments. This often comes up during a relaxation pose when it might be difficult to settle down. Cueing might include "Please be quiet and respect your fellow classmates' relaxation time."

The nurturing environment of yoga emulates the principle of friendship. To set the tone for friendship, you can state, "This is a place where we are all friends." This could be facilitated with younger students by starting class in a circle, with students holding hands and saying aloud, "Hands are for helping and never hurting" or "This is a place where everyone is special and listened to with respect." Another nice closing activity with the younger students is for them to find another student and pay him or her a sincere compliment.

With older students, a nurturing environment can be created by encouraging peer dialogue, which should always be positive and supportive in tone. With older students, having rules that establish the groundwork for a yoga class can help set the correct environment, such as entering the yoga class silently and sitting quietly and not chatting. It is always helpful to recognize and acknowledge any class by thanking them for desirable behaviors such as listening, helping, saying thank you, waiting for their turns, and so on.

If students experience conflict with each other, they need to know it is their responsibility to deal with conflict in a constructive and positive way. This may not be modeled in today's society, where disrespecting and blaming others is commonplace. One way to communicate a different opinion is to use "I" messages, which help students clearly state what is wrong, how they feel, and what they want. An example is "I felt left out and sad when you walked away, and I would appreciate it if you listened to what I have to say." This replaces a "you" statement—"You are a jerk for leaving me out, and you always do that"—where the emphasis is on blame and putting the other person on the defensive.

Try as much as possible to let students work out their conflicts with one another. Avoid jumping into and taking sides in a conflict. Remaining calm and identifying the problem without blaming will help set the correct tone. Whatever the problem is, the climate of yoga is always win–win, meaning students are working together against the problem and not against each other.

TEACHING TECHNIQUES FOR YOGA

There may not be a lot of opportunity in a student's life for the safe and nurturing space yoga can provide. This section provides ideas for teaching techniques that include managing the yoga class, rules and discipline, and safety. A critical aspect in managing the class, setting rules and discipline, and maintaining safety is deciding what will make the yoga experience enjoyable for all.

Managing the Yoga Classroom

You can use several methods to foster better class management.

1. In proximity reinforcement, you walk around the class to reinforce listening and on-task behavior by standing close to a student who might be distracting the group. Another method is to stand with your back to the wall so all students can see. This allows the students to follow you doing the pose.

2. Demonstration can sometimes encourage correct form. You can ask older students to stop and watch how to do a pose and then go back to their spaces to try the pose.

3. Inclusive circle is another class organizational method where all participants are in a circle. This means no one is standing behind another and not able to see or getting lost in the back of the room. You are part of the circle, not in the middle.

4. Another strategy is putting students in pairs or groups. You can quickly divide the class by birthdays or color of the shirts they are wearing so friends don't always work together and certain children are not always left out and alone. Dividing students up by gender is not recommended. The boys versus the girls, or competing teams for that matter, is not part of yoga's philosophy.

Structuring a Yoga Class

Structure can provide comfort for students by their knowing each yoga session will have consistent rules, sequence, and structure. Structure in yoga should not be approached as rigid and authoritative but as a way to add form to the yoga practice that is comforting and enjoyable. Students look forward to the natural progression that structure provides. Routines need to be consistent and be taught, practiced, and reviewed with students. There should be a procedure for entering the yoga space, leaving the yoga space, using equipment, and using the bathroom or getting water. Class should have a beginning and ending ritual. Providing a way for students to make a smooth and natural transition from what they were doing before coming to yoga and then back to the next task or activity is important. The beginning and ending are often what students comment on as their favorite part of yoga class.

There are several methods to start and end a class, and specific chapters in this book address beginning and ending class in more detail. To provide you with just a brief idea for structure, typically the class will begin with getting out the yoga mats and sitting down on them or coming into the center of the room and finding a place to sit in the circle. This could be followed by a breathing exercise or a poem or short story to set the theme for that day's lesson. What follows is similar to a typical physical activity class: a warm-up, a workout phase, and a cool-down phase. This structure allows for the most physiological and psychological benefits to be obtained. In yoga there is a more-natural ebb and flow to the sequence, allowing for rest periods and reflection between more-active poses. This allows for a way to show students they can work hard but need to balance effort with restoration. Rest periods might include poses that are restorative or restful or simply lying quietly. The workout phase may include poses or yoga games that incorporate the poses just learned depending on the age of the group you are working with.

For example, a 30-minute class for elementary school students might have the following structure:

1. Introductory activities: 3 minutes for a breathing exercise followed by a story that sets a theme for the day's class

2. Warm-up poses: 4 minutes

3. Standing poses: 5 minutes

4. Games: 8 minutes

5. Cool-down poses: 4 minutes

6. Relaxation poses: 3 minutes

7. Closing transition activity: reflective circle. Question: How can we all be a better friend? 3 minutes

If you have less than 30 minutes, you can shorten some activities, but it is recommended to always have an opening breathing exercise and closing relaxation segment for all yoga classes. Remember that these are just general guidelines—yoga does not need to have a regimented and formal timetable. Pay attention to the students' energy and keep the intention of moderation and balance.

Scheduling yoga class will probably be a factor of finding time in busy school schedules. Some schools have adopted Friday afternoons as yoga time each week. It is hard to do yoga directly after a meal, but yoga classes may need to be scheduled right after "Friday pizza" in the cafeteria. This may prove to be a teachable moment, when a discussion about healthy eating might work well. Normally it is suggested to eat something easy to digest (such as fruit) before class, not to eat a heavy meal 2 to 3 hours before class, and to eat a light snack and hydrate after class. Ask participants to throw away gum before class because it interferes with breathing, and snapping gum is a surefire distraction.

Handling Embarrassing Moments

Gas. There, it has been said. Often in class, participants get gas. A chorus of giggles and comments happen. At this time, ignore it and move on. At a later time, this could be a teachable moment about the importance of paying attention to the fuel put into the body and how to best take care of the body—all important lessons in yoga and life. It is natural to have gas, especially if students are eating the diets rich in fiber, vegetables, and fruit that we are encouraging them to eat. Students can be encouraged to find foods that agree with their individual digestion. We do not pay a whole lot of attention to digestion and assume stomachaches are normal.

Setting Rules

What rules to apply depends on the individual instructor and the class situation (e.g., a class taught in a yoga studio differs from yoga taught in a classroom setting). In general, the rules should convey the importance of respecting all participants' personal space, not distracting from others' learning experiences, keeping voices and language respectful, and listening to the teacher and other students.

Try to keep rules very simple and basic, such as the following:

- Be respectful.
- Be positive.
- Be safe.

Be consistent and fair as much as possible, and allow each student to start each class with a clean slate. For example, a student who may have been a distraction last class may need to be reminded of the parameters for participating in yoga class but starts this class with a fresh start. Just as each yoga experience is a chance to start with a beginner's mind, each class should be taken with this attitude. Encourage students to take responsibility for their own movements and actions. This also means their movements and actions never interfere with the safety of their teacher or fellow yogis.

Another important intention of all students is to be positive. "Yes, I can" needs to be the mantra and the attitude taken when students start to belittle themselves or each other or become negative about the yoga class. It is important to redirect and remind students to be positive and follow this rule. Rules will need to be reviewed often. Posting the rules in the yoga space and printing them in a flyer for parents to review with their children are other ideas.

Providing Discipline

In yoga, the general atmosphere is always positive, and the instructor should always make comments that reinforce appropriate behavior. For example, if a student is distracting and not getting ready for class to start, you could say, "You can join the circle when you are ready by sitting on your unfolded mat." The tendency might be to point out that what the student is doing is wrong, but rewording statements to emphasize the positive benefits of correct actions sets the correct tone. However, there may be times when discipline must be applied. Again, the instructor's individual comfort and teaching style will dictate the discipline necessary. In physical education classes or academic classes, discipline might be telling a student to leave the room for a time-out, for example. Nevertheless, inclusion is paramount. The following is an example of enforcing discipline without exclusion.

■ Step 1: Offer a friendly reminder. Stating the student's name, say, "This is a friendly reminder to please remember our yoga rules."

■ Step 2: Give a verbal warning. For example, "Stop, think, make a better choice. Step off the mat, and take some time for yourself."

■ Step 3: Announce consequences, perhaps losing a privilege that the student has been given such as helping lead the ending of the class or being the yoga assistant. Here is an example: "You will need to regroup, refocus, and return when you are ready to do yoga" or "You will need to leave the yoga space if I need to speak with you again."

■ Step 4: Deliver consequences. A student may need to leave her yoga space. There may be a designated space in the room where the students go to reflect and develop a plan for change before they can return to the yoga space. In cases where the student breaks a rule that involves another student, such as making fun of someone or calling someone a name, it is the student's responsibility: You broke it, you fix it. The student would then need to apologize before rejoining the group.

It would be unfortunate to exclude a student from yoga. Yoga is hopefully fun and valued as a special activity. However, there may be times when a student needs to be told he can participate again only when he is ready to take responsibility for his yoga and respect the yoga practice of others, including the teacher.

The kind of language used in class should always build trust. For example, in a situation where several 4th-grade students are pushing each other trying to get a yoga mat, the first inclination might be to yell at them to knock it off. To build trust, your response might include the following: "When we participate in yoga without pushing each other, we can all be safe. I want you all to be safe. How can we make this space safe?" By asking questions, students problem-solve for themselves. Again, it might be easier to tell the students the correct response, but by putting the initiative on them, there will be long-lasting results for classroom management and discipline.

Providing Safety

Incorporating the methods mentioned for classroom management and the rituals for proper conduction of the class addresses many safety issues. Yoga is a safe physical activity, as there are always ways to adapt a task for a student. The constant goal is to progress from simple to complex and to adjust each activity to fit a wide range of student abilities. It is important to know if your students have any health problems or accessibility needs. Accessibility means providing extra accommodations to any student who might need it. An example of this is a student who comes to yoga class in a wheelchair. This is not a problem in yoga because the poses can be adapted to the wheelchair. There is more information on adapting yoga to wheelchairs or chairs in the resource section.

Teaching Styles

In teaching the whole child, our methods of teaching need to vary so we can engage as many different styles of learning as possible. The traditional command method of teaching has the instructor standing in front of the students and demonstrating the skill, with the students following. This method does help students get a quick idea of the skill, but it doesn't allow for exploration or consider the individual needs of the students. It may be helpful to explore the following additional methods when teaching yoga.

- **Task**—A student might be asked to independently come up with a pose or change a pose to make it take on a different quality. Setting up stations where students spend a specific amount of time practicing a specific pose and then moving on to the next station is an example of the task method.

- **Reciprocal**—Students work cooperatively in pairs and give each other feedback.

- **Self-check**—The students might have a checklist of aspects of an activity they are doing. For example, in the relaxation segment, there might be a list of five progressive steps the students go through to get ready for relaxation.

- **Inclusion**—The students are given several options and choose the options they wish to do. For example in instructing tree pose, where a student stands (the supporting leg like a tree trunk) on one foot (the foot like roots of the tree) (see figure 3.2), there are several options. These options include resting the other foot on top of the supporting foot, placing the sole of the other foot against the calf, or for more difficulty, placing the foot against the inner thigh. The next level of difficulty would be giving options for the upper body, such as holding onto a chair; placing the hands on the hips, then on the shoulders; or moving the arms from straight out to the sides to overhead and gently swaying in the breeze.

- **Exploratory**—The students are given the opportunity to find a single correct response to a task (called a convergent task) or multiple responses to a task (called a divergent task). An example of a convergent task is for students to find their best way to stand strong and tall on the ground with both feet. Through their own exploration, the students are doing the mountain pose, which is an important stepping-stone to other standing and balance poses that require a strong foundation (see figure 3.3). An example of a divergent task is asking the students to find as many different ways to balance, thus inviting them to balance on their hands, on their bottoms, or on one foot.

- **Problem solving and guided discovery**—The students are given a problem to solve alone, in pairs, or in a group. A problem or question can be posed: "Do you know what balance is? Put yourself in the most balanced position you can. Now find a way to be a little less balanced. Find a way to be the least balanced."

- **Challenge**—The students are given a challenge such as creating and naming a pose with a partner.

Using the Voice

The use of the voice, the words to help students learn, and the ability to keep students focused are important elements of teaching yoga, so observe the level and tone of voice you use. The use of voice sets the tone: Yoga is fun, but the voice needs to be loud enough so everyone hears and understands. Try to speak from the belly and not the throat, with a soothing and nurturing quality. Take time to pause to let students absorb what has been said. Often a novice instructor will provide too much information; it is better to keep instructions as simple as possible. It will be necessary to repeat instructions several times or break them down into parts. When teaching a standing pose, for example, first introduce the placement of the lower body, and then add the upper body later on. Check often for understanding, and try to find another or simpler way of explaining. The voice will change with the transitions to relaxation, where it may become softer and quieter to facilitate quiet and respite.

Cueing

Cues should always encourage students to become more mindful and to pay attention to their own bodies, emotions, and sensations. Using language that emphasizes the concept of feeling can help facilitate this. Examples include "Feel the earth support you as you stand tall" and "Feel your breath deep and slow in your belly as you practice this pose."

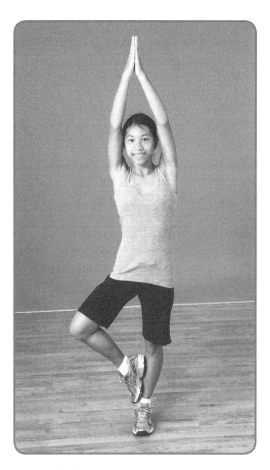

FIGURE 3.2   Tree pose.

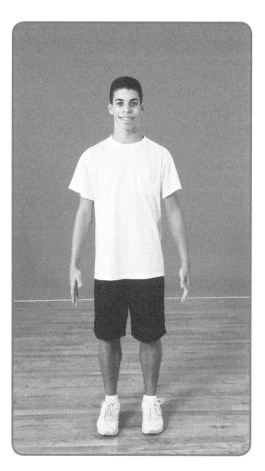

FIGURE 3.3   Mountain pose.

Language

Using language that encourages exploration and problem solving is another way to guide students, such as "How many ways can you . . ." "Discover ways you can . . ." "Notice if . . .?" The following are other examples of motivating cues: "Can you make your pose softer or lighter?" "Can you grow your spine like a sunflower reaching to the sun?" "Can you blow up a big balloon in your belly while you play with this pose?" "How many different ways can you move your arms?" With practice and observation, an instructor will naturally find many ways to help cue students. Also by having her own yoga practice, an instructor can experientially explore poses herself and provide insight to her students in turn.

Using Inclusive Language

The climate of a class needs to focus on student-centered learning, and providing cues that guide the students to focus on finding what is best for them encourages this. Inclusive language means opening up your instruction to include multiple senses that encourage learning through multiple learning styles. Using inclusive language is the part of teaching that allows for a lot of creativity. For example, when we hear the word *visualization*, we might imagine a huge screen in the brain and focus only on visual images. This is one method of teaching, but we can also incorporate guided imagination. This is where detail is added to make use of the other senses to make the "image" more rich and detailed. Asking students to use their own imagination adds to this, including the senses of feeling, touching, tasting, smelling, and hearing. Here is an example: "Imagine that a large magnet on the top of your head is reaching to the metal beam in the ceiling overhead. The magnet pulls your whole spine upward, and you feel your neck getting longer and longer."

Another way to be inclusive is to use a vocabulary that is inclusive to all—not just people who have a previous understanding of yoga. Yoga is not a religion. It is a method for healthy and balanced living that supports common humanistic values. Yoga has been misinterpreted to be a religious practice, and parents might therefore be hesitant to let their children participate. Yoga gives children the time and experiences to seek answers within themselves, to find their own wisdom that has been laid within the foundation of their own family values. The following are suggested words that will help best support communicating the wisdom of yoga to your students. Instead of perhaps *meditation*, the phrases *reflection time, understanding time*, or *calming time* can be used. Instead of the word *spirit*, try *silence, stillness, peace, quiet*, or *stepping inside of yourself*. In yoga, the use of the hands in the prayer position over the heart space may not be appropriate for all learners. Putting both hands one over the other over the heart space, symbolizing a "strong and safe place to feel centered," could be substituted. If at any time you do not feel comfortable with any of the cues or words presented here or in any yoga text or class, feel free to substitute language that is more appropriate and sensitive to your needs and the needs of the students.

Including Language Learners

You may have English as a Second Language (ESL) students in your classes. Keeping language simple is one way to help ESL students learn, as well as giving students pictures of the poses to look at. See the resource section for visual aid sources.

Focusing Students

One of the most valuable tools in yoga is helping students tune out distractions and stay on task and focused. As stated previously, cues that emphasize paying attention to oneself and not others help create focus. Another method is called dhristi, or focus spot. Dhristi is a specific eye focal point used to develop focus and concentration. As a general rule, the eyes should gaze in the direction of the stretch. An example of a cue for dhristi is "Find a spot on the floor ahead, and keep the eyes gently glued to this spot during the balance poses." A dhristi aid can be introduced, such as a Beanie Baby or any object the students can keep their eyes focused on. Remind students that if performing dhristi ever bothers the neck (e.g., when looking up at the ceiling), they can drop the eye gaze to the floor. Shutting the eyes may be thought of as a way to focus, but by keeping the eyes open with a steady, relaxed gaze, students learn to tune out distractions. For example, when driving we can't close our eyes, but we can calm the breath and keep our eyes focused to deal with a traffic jam.

Providing Feedback

Positive reinforcement should be the hallmark of teaching, with praise and positive corrections and maximum participation in every learning task. It is often easier to point out to students what they are doing wrong than to provide feedback on what they are doing right and suggestions for improvement. A student should never be singled out if he is not holding his arms correctly, for instance, but a comment can be made to the whole class, such as "Remember to keep your arms strong and like arrows coming out from your shoulders." Feedback needs to be meaningful and not just idle chatter. The feedback must be of value to the learner and not about the instructor. An example is "You must be very proud of your effort in yoga today" instead of "I am very proud of your yoga effort today."

The more specific the feedback, the better it will reinforce learning. Specific feedback needs to be stated in a neutral voice that is factual and descriptive without judging. An example of specific feedback is "When we do the tree pose, we stand firm and strong on one foot, with our eyes on our focus point." Remember to provide feedback that not only focuses on the muscles used but also includes information about feelings or sensations, such as "Think of your whole body during sun salutation soaking in the strength and energy from the sun," "Be sure to keep your knees slightly bent, or soft," and "Great job of keeping your legs strong and your eyes focused during this balance pose."

In teaching yoga, some behaviors just need to be ignored, and feedback only fuels incorrect behavior. An example is a student purposely doing the pose incorrectly. The rest of the class will probably continue to follow your instructions. Unless safety is an issue, ignore the student; she will probably give up since she is not getting any attention drawn to her.

Providing Feedback by Assisting Students

An assist is when an instructor uses her hands to assist or correct a student while he is doing a pose. You might touch a student lightly between the shoulder blades to remind him to keep them together as a form of feedback. Appropriate and respectful touching needs to be introduced, and you need to ask permission before touching a student with a statement such as "Can I give you some guidance to help you relax in this pose?" However, physical touching may not be appropriate in teaching your students. To provide tactile cues, a student could stand against a wall while doing a standing pose such as mountain in order to feel the back of the head, the shoulder blades, and the gluteals touch the wall as feedback to make her aware of her posture and how it feels to stand up straight.

CONSTRUCTING CREATIVE YOGA EXPERIENCES

Creating motivating learning experiences is part of the art of teaching. This section will hopefully spark your creative flame. With more experience, you will cultivate a host of experiences to enrich the students' yoga practice.

Finding the Best Yoga Space

Creating a nurturing and inviting yoga space is an important aspect of teaching yoga. In reality, very limited space is available in most schools and facilities. Keep an open mind, and remember that yoga does not need a great deal of space. Desks can be moved aside in the classroom, or if the time for yoga is not very long, students can do their poses right next to their desks. The following are some general recommendations for choosing a yoga space and equipment.

1. Have enough space so students can move freely while on their yoga mats and so the mats are not stepped on if students are moving around the room. A yoga mat measures 6 feet by 2 feet (1.8 meters by .6 meter).

2. Use a room that provides natural light, with a way to regulate the temperature and lights. The room should provide adequate ventilation so students have fresh air and do not get overheated. The room temperature should be kept on the comfortably warm side, and if the room is cold, space heaters can be used to bring the temperature up.

3. Dimming the lights can encourage quiet and relaxation time. Lights can also be used to cue students: "When the lights flicker, it is time to quiet down and go back to your yoga mats."

4. The flooring should be easily cleaned and resistant to slipping and sliding. Carpeted floors are difficult to clean on a regular basis, but they do provide some cushioning. Wood floors are often seen in recreational facilities that have exercise rooms; these floors are easy to clean, but caution is needed as they can be slippery when wet. The area should be kept as clean as possible, and students should be encouraged and expected to respect the cleanliness of the yoga space.

5. The room should be in a quiet area without a lot of traffic and distractions and with the ability to minimize interruptions such as an intercom, TV, phones, and clutter. Cell phones should be shut off, as even the vibrate mode can be distracting.

Any room can be transformed into a yoga space by hanging colorful banners, student artwork, or inspirational posters. Keep yoga props such as music instruments, scarves, Beanie Babies, and blocks in colorful laundry baskets or storage containers. Blankets can provide warmth during relaxation time. Colorful Mexican blankets are inexpensive, are durable, and can be easily washed.

Using Yoga Equipment

Yoga is a terrific activity for most schools because it does not require a lot of equipment or space. The best kind of activity mat for yoga is called a sticky mat. This mat allows the participant to move on a skid-free surface. Exercise mats and wrestling mats are not recommended, as they can easily move and are too soft to provide a solid foundation for most yoga poses. If possible, participants should purchase their own mats for sanitary reasons. Having their own mats at home may even encourage practicing yoga outside of class time. If the mats are used by various students, they can be wiped down with a gentle cleaner that is nontoxic, as some students have sensitivities to strong-smelling cleaners. Mats can also be put in the washing machine and line dried. Mat material can be bought in bulk and cut into 5- to 6-foot (1.5 to 1.8 meter) lengths (see the resources for wholesale resources). If the class is taking place in a carpeted room, having mats may not be necessary, although caution should be taken as sliding can still happen on carpet. Having some kind of a designated individual space such as a carpet square can be useful when teaching in a carpeted area.

During yoga practice, a lot of heat is created, and a towel can come in handy to wipe sweaty hands. A towel can also be used as a prop or a helping tool. For example, in the forward stretch where one sits with both legs stretched out in the front, the towel can be placed around the bottom of the feet; holding onto the ends of the towel can encourage a deeper stretch. An athletic towel that measures 24 by 12 inches (60 by 30 centimeters) is recommended over a beach or bath towel, which is bulky and cumbersome to use.

Music can be used to greet students, set the tone or a theme for class, and expose students to different music from other cultures. There are tremendous resources for music (see the resources section). A CD of various songs can be put together to help pace the class. Different tempos can be used for active poses and relaxing music for cool-down poses and final relaxation. The research points to acoustical music without words as being the best for relaxation (Synder & Chlan, 1999). Students can be encouraged to bring in their own music. Finding music that students might not encounter normally can enrich their experience—try the Beatles! A chime or bell can be used at the start of class and to finish after relaxation as a nurturing way to signal in-class transitions.

At the end of class, you can provide "eye pillows" (covered with a tissue to keep them sanitary) to aid students in relaxing and quieting down. Eye pillows can be easily made of colorful scrap cotton fabric sewn into 4- by 8-inch (10 by 20 centimeter) rectangles filled with rice or buckwheat (see figure 3.4). Beanie Babies also make nice eye pillows (see figure 3.5).

Although there is a whole industry of yoga workout clothes, whatever is comfortable for students to wear is fine. Street clothes are not recommended, as jeans and belts can constrict movement. Baggy clothes interfere with the ability to assess

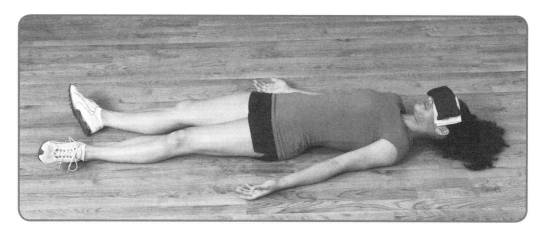

FIGURE 3.4 Eye pillow.

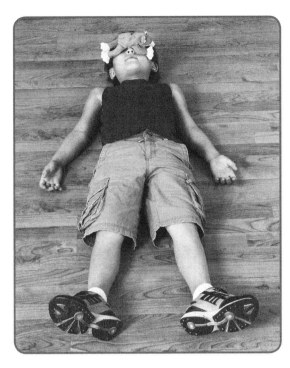

FIGURE 3.5   Beanie Baby eye pillow.

alignment (e.g., a student could be locking her knees and it would be difficult to see this). A baggy T-shirt may get in the way of breathing during inversion (upside down) poses. Yoga attire should not be distracting to others. Most schools have dress codes for physical education, and those same guidelines can be used for yoga. You can also recommend appropriate attire for the yoga class and gently advise any students if their attire is distracting.

Females can wear shorts or yoga pants that are cut closer to the body than sweat pants, with a tank top or a closer-fitting T-shirt or athletic shirt. Males can also wear shorts or athletic pants with a closer-fitting athletic top. Students can wear layers of clothing, as the temperature of the body will rise. In yoga, the core temperature of the body increases, thereby facilitating stretching, decreasing pain, and improving circulation. When the lesson moves into the cool-down poses and relaxation, students can put on a hooded sweatshirt and use the hood to cover their faces to block out light for relaxation.

Personal cleanliness is essential. Part of yoga etiquette and practice is for students to know they should wear clean clothes to yoga class, not sweaty clothes stored in the locker for weeks on end. It is also vital for students to consider not wearing overpowering deodorants, colognes, and perfumes, as other participants may have sensitivities and allergies. Jewelry such as watches, large hoop earrings, or heavy pendants may interfere with the poses and should be removed.

It is customary not to wear street shoes into the yoga classroom or space, so shoes should be removed before entering the class. A yoga studio or space is considered a special place or sanctuary, and wearing shoes with street dirt is not conducive to keeping the space clean and nurturing. However, this may not be logistically possible in many school situations because there is no designated space for yoga. But asking students to remove their shoes and having a broom or sweeper handy might help keep the space clean. Yoga is traditionally practiced in bare feet for safety, as stocking feet will easily slip. Practicing in bare feet also helps strengthen the feet and improve sense of balance. Participants may experience foot cramps as the feet get stronger, and this is normal. Sometimes with older students, taking off their shoes in public becomes an issue. Bringing in a pair of clean athletic shoes might be a way to compromise.

It is important to find your own comfort level for distractions, such as when a student needs to leave class to get a sip of water or use the bathroom. Water bottles can help maintain hydration, and it is necessary to remind students to hydrate during and after class. Taking a water break during the class can help keep students hydrated. Another way might be to establish a rule such as allowing students to get water one time during class and then quietly return to their yoga space.

Using Props

All kinds of interesting and creative equipment can be part of the yoga toolbox. Musical instruments such as shakers, drums, cymbals, bells, and sound sticks can be used. Gather up whatever you can find in the physical education storeroom such as hoops, jump ropes, scooters, tennis balls, ping pong balls, and soft (Nerf) balls. Make a trip to the dollar store to find balloons, scarves, ribbons, Beanie Babies, and bubbles.

A variety of specific yoga props are also available, such as soft blocks and blankets to help in trying a posture. A chair or a wall may be necessary in order to allow for adaptation and achieving some

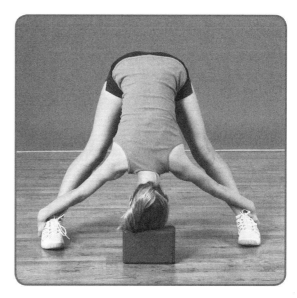

FIGURE 3.6 Standing wide-angle pose with yoga block.

success in a posture. In the tree pose, for example, the wall could provide tactile cues as to a person's posture, alignment, and sense of security against falling. When those postures evolve with the gaining of strength and balance, then the props can be slowly removed. Another way to use yoga props is putting the hands or head on a yoga block instead of straining to reach the floor as demonstrated in the standing wide-angle pose seen in figure 3.6. Each yoga class can be unique by working with creative variations in instruction methods, the environment, and the equipment.

Connecting Yoga to Healthy and Balanced Living

Yoga for healthy and balanced living has as its foundation the goal of using the lessons from yoga to add to the quality of our students' learning and everyday lives. As mentioned previously, yoga is not a stringing together of poses but a way to infuse learning into a physical, emotional, and social activity. One way to do this is to include "reflection time" at the close of class. This can be done by sitting in a circle and asking each student to share something he learned in yoga class that day or what makes him thankful or happy. Older students could write a positive affirmation or intention or a journal entry about their yoga experience for that day. Although the purpose of journal writing is never to force ideas or demand the writing be done in any particular way, students can have a tendency to simply report what happened in class. Instead of asking the students to report back, encourage them to reflect on how yoga affects them on different levels, such as feelings, thoughts, and reactions. Examples of reflection exercises are open-ended statements such as "I learned . . . today," "I felt . . . today," or "I was concerned about . . . today." The class may have had a theme or an intention statement, such as gratitude, forgiveness, or being still and listening to your own voice, and you may ask students to reflect on that theme. Creative writing or drawing or any art form can be a wonderful way to finish class by leaving enough time after relaxation to just enjoy writing, coloring, or drawing.

Another way to bring yoga into the students' lives is to ask parents to participate in some of the yoga exercises. A pose of the day can be sent home with the students to teach their families. Both the students and their families can keep a gratitude journal by writing down five things they are grateful for each day. Families could set an intention each morning, see what happens as the day unfolds, and discuss their experience each evening at family dinner. To incorporate the concept of karma yoga—service to others—families can volunteer together to "pay it forward" by adopting a family in need, doing errands or chores for a neighbor, cleaning a park, collecting food items, or doing whatever their community needs. Offer special events such as a special yoga class for parents and their children to practice together. An entry fee of a canned food or nonperishable item could be collected and donated to a local food bank.

Teaching Suggestions for Specific Age Groups

Creating great yoga classes offers the challenge of finding ways to connect to students' unique learning styles. No matter what the age of the students, yoga classes should be inclusive, individualized, and enjoyable. In working with children, it is important to remember that their development is age related but not age specific, meaning there can be a wide variation in the development of children of the same age. Each student will have a unique and dynamic timetable for her developmental growth. You will notice a wide range of differences between students depending on the specific skill or movement, heredity and physical characteristics, and previous experience.

Understanding Developmental Milestones

The developmental milestone chart (see table 3.1 on page 42) offers a general idea of what children of specific ages should be able to do physically, cognitively, and psychosocially in your yoga classes. Many of the physical developmental milestones are naturally part of yoga. Watch a baby put his toes in his mouth and you will know how the pose happy baby, which is lying on the back holding onto the toes with the hands, got its name. Young babies practice yoga as they naturally learn through movement. For example, the cobra pose is done lying facedown, bringing the legs together like the tail of a snake, and lifting the chest off the floor with the arms. This developmental movement is the stepping-stone that all infants do to develop the trunk control needed as a precursor for creeping.

Countless components of movement can be incorporated into classes and poses. Learning about movement occurs on different levels.

■ **Body movement**—The first level of learning is how the body moves. Starting at this first level, there are three ways the body can move: locomotor, nonlocomotor, and manipulative.

1. Locomotor movement allows for moving around an area and includes eight basic movements: walk, run, gallop, slide, jump, hop, leap, and skip. Locomotor skills are influenced by the student's age, lower-body strength, balance, and neurological development.

2. Nonlocomotor, or axial, movement includes 14 stationary movements: bending, stretching, twisting, turning, pushing, pulling, rising, collapsing, swinging, swaying, dodging, spinning, shaking, and balancing.

3. Manipulation is the final movement, where the hands or the feet use equipment to perform fine motor and gross motor skills. Fine motor skills use the hands and fingers and include tying shoelaces, using scissors, or writing. Gross motor skills use the large muscles of the legs and arms and are skills used primarily in games and sports such as rolling, kicking, or dribbling.

These three ways of moving the body can be combined by using dance steps or sport skill movement patterns such as a basketball layup in yoga class. Be creative and think outside the box to find fun and imaginative ways to include what students gravitate toward in yoga. Perhaps try a hip-hop theme infused with yoga poses.

■ **Body awareness**—The second level of understanding movement is body awareness. Body awareness includes transfer of body weight, balance, flight, making various shapes, and eye focus. Activities in yoga class to improve body awareness could include making the shapes of the alphabet with the body or doing a jumping jack and then freezing into a pose.

■ **Space**—The third level of movement includes an awareness of space (spatial), including personal space and general space. Personal space can be explored in yoga by asking students to stretch out on their own mats without touching others; the concept of general space can be taught by asking students to move to the music anywhere in the yoga room without bumping anyone or anything. Learning the different directions of movement (e.g., forward, backward, sideways, up, and down) as well as sizes (e.g., giant or small) are also included in teaching spatial awareness. Finally, the various pathways of movement such as straight, curved, and zigzag as well as the levels of low, medium, and high are aspects of spatial awareness.

■ **Movement quality**—Level four of understanding movement describes the different qualities of movement. The quality of time involves moving quickly, moving slowly, accelerating or decelerating, and moving to a basic beat or rhythm. The quality of effort includes movement that is strong, firm, light, or soft. Here is an example: "Tiptoe quietly, and when you hear the drum beat, freeze into the [_____] pose and become strong and firm. . . . That is great. The next time you hear the drum, melt your pose down into the floor and become relaxed and soft."

■ **Environment**—The final aspect of learning how movement takes place is in relationship to the surrounding environment. The environment can include the relationship with space (e.g., moving near or far); the relationship of body parts to other body parts (e.g., raising the arms from the sides of the body up overhead during a balancing pose); and the relationship with others (e.g., playing follow the leader or skipping around with a partner).

These dynamic levels of movement need to be taught while considering your students' readiness, motivation, and opportunity to practice. The following pages provide some suggestions incorporating these considerations when teaching yoga to specific age groups.

Teaching Preschool Yoga

In preschool, the emphasis is on imagination and how bodies move and work. In early childhood (ages 3 to 5), the emphasis is on fundamental motor skills, with the primary goal of establishing a positive attitude about movement and appreciation of the importance of participation in lifelong activity. To integrate motor, cognitive, emotional, and social development, providing a variety of opportunities for both individual and cooperative play is necessary. Maximum participation is important, but also keep in mind this group needs rest as well. Games such as duck, duck, goose do not allow maximum participation. In this game, students sit passively and watch other students get picked to play. It is not that taking turns is not an important concept for this age group, but this game does not provide maximum participation and inclusion and therefore is not effective pedagogy.

TABLE 3.1 Developmental Milestones

Grade	Movement benchmarks	Yoga benchmarks	Cognitive domain	Affective domain
Pre-K-2	▪ Coordination of gross motor and fine motor skills ▪ Starting and stopping on signal ▪ Moving through environment with body control ▪ Traveling different pathways ▪ Starting to learn body control	▪ Making different shapes at different levels ▪ Moving to music in different directions and at different levels; freezing into a specific pose when music stops ▪ Relaxed breathing	▪ Clapping to the beat of music ▪ Reciting the different levels and directions they can move in ▪ Verbalizing various elements of movements or poses ▪ Applying problem solving to simple movement challenges ▪ Responding to cues	▪ Using movement as a way to communicate and express themselves ▪ Achieving a sense of self-satisfaction from expressive movement ▪ Enjoying moving to music ▪ Able to keep still and quiet for short periods of time
3-5	▪ Jumping rope ▪ Throwing and catching a ball; dribbling a ball ▪ Fundamental movement: locomotor, nonlocomotor, and manipulative ▪ Following dance sequence to rhythm of the music	▪ Combining several poses ▪ Exploring and adapting fundamental movement skills, with a variety of poses in a dynamic environment	▪ Verbally counting to the beat of music ▪ Analyzing and providing feedback on a yoga pose to a partner ▪ Verbally describing a simple yoga pose ▪ Knowing the history of yoga on a knowledge test	▪ Taking turns appropriately ▪ Can select partners ▪ Obeying rules and class etiquette ▪ Can work cooperatively with a partner making a pose
6-8	▪ Wide variation in maturation levels: emphasis on physical development but with options so all can be successful ▪ Able to perform fundamental movement skills in combinations of open and closed environments	▪ Emphasis on strong posture and correct body mechanics while doing poses and pose sequences	▪ Encouraging the why behind concepts by promoting creative thinking and problem solving ▪ Promoting leadership and cooperative learning ▪ Emphasis on physical activity throughout the life span	▪ Need positive social interaction ▪ Need strategies for emotional control and stress management ▪ Can be critical of adults and want independence ▪ Need to understand responsibility and importance of rules ▪ Competitive and will need to understand yoga is not competitive
9-12	▪ Able to do adult-style yoga (there can be wide variations in ability among individual students)	▪ Able to do adult-style yoga	▪ Able to form and verbalize opinions ▪ Able to use logic and analysis	▪ Tend to want things immediately; impulsive ▪ Feel indestructible ▪ Can be moody, and emotions can be overwhelming at times

Make sure to have enough equipment for all that includes a variety of shapes, sizes, textures, and weights. This group can benefit from a lot of nontraditional equipment such as scarves and balloons. Using fun music, singing songs, and using puppets and books are terrific ways to motivate this age group. With this age group, practice through repetition is important while exploring visual, kinesthetic, and auditory opportunities for learning.

The following are some things to keep in mind when working with preschool students:

- Compliment good behavior.
- Encourage asking of questions.
- Provide opportunities to make choices.
- Encourage expressing emotions in appropriate ways.
- Use time-outs when students display unacceptable behavior.
- Be consistent and firm.

With all age groups, but particularly with younger students, it is vital to notice the cues they give you about their energy and attention. Having this age group do brief periods of activity while building in time to rest and recover and repetition (practice) will allow them to reap the benefits of yoga participation.

Teaching Primary Elementary School Yoga: Grades K-2

In this age group, we continue to build the fundamental movement skills, and the various aspects of gross motor movement begin. The emphasis is on traveling in various pathways, moving at different levels, and starting and stopping and body control. Developing fine motor movement begins at this age as well. In psychosocial skill development, the goal is learning cooperation and responsible behavior.

The following are some things to keep in mind when working with primary elementary school students:

- This is a very optimistic age—always keep the students' energy positive.
- Imagination and play need to be the focus—it may not look like yoga, but if it is imaginative, fun, and student centered, it is!

Teaching Upper Elementary School Yoga: Grades 3-5

The use of partners and group cooperative activities can inspire this age group, and they are very responsive to these kinds of activities. However, these students are very aware of individual differences (i.e., who is the best and who is the worst). Reinforcing the importance of individual differences and not competition is critical here. Peer pressure starts to become an important factor with this age group. Setting guidelines on how to deal with peer pressure both in and out of the class is an important skill for this group, such as dealing with conflict and understanding other points of view. In class, you need to expect that rules will be followed, and being consistent and firm with the rules is necessary when working with upper elementary students.

With this age group, it is also important to emphasize self-care and respect for personal boundaries. For example, in yoga we respect others' space by moving only on our own yoga mats. In yoga for this age group, you need to pace the class, as they have a tendency to push and overdo it. Asking students to pay attention to their minds and bodies and mixing physical activity with rest is vital as well.

The following are some things to keep in mind when working with upper elementary school students:

- Compliment cooperation as much as possible.
- Encourage students to be open about their feelings.
- Infuse reading as much as possible.

Teaching Middle School Yoga: Grades 6-8

This age group will be very diverse in terms of their physical, intellectual, and social development, with the added complexities of the transition from childhood to young adulthood. This group tends to be self-absorbed and can become confused and moody. The goal is to help them be physically active and achieve individual success. By providing several levels of a task as guided choices, the environment will be safe and inclusive for all.

These students want to be talked to as equals, and they respond well to caring adults. Positive socialization is paramount with this age group. This group needs to cooperate and communicate with each other and honor the strengths and differences they all bring to class. Students will generally be cooperative and considerate but at times can be unpredictable and inconsistent. They can also be rebellious and critical of themselves and others. When there is conflict, they need to work to resolve it themselves as much as possible. With this age group, being fair and consistent is critical, as is having students take responsibility for their own behavior. This age group needs guidance with being self-aware while at the same time respecting others. As stated previously in the section on setting rules, making sure this age group's attitude and language are positive is critical. Nothing can drag a group down more than having a student or a group of students disrespect a yoga activity.

During adolescence, female students can mature up to 2 years before males, with rapid spurts in growth and the development of secondary sexual characteristics including fat distribution, breasts, pubic hair, and the start of menstruation. Doing yoga poses before and during menstruation can help bring balance to the body. Any strenuous poses may be done for shorter periods of time or leave the student the option of finding restorative poses.

The onset of secondary sexual characteristics will vary widely among both genders, which can be a great source of anxiety. This age group has a preoccupation with appearance. With this preoccupation comes a possibility of disordered eating patterns, such as restrictive dieting, or use of diet pills. Also keep in mind there will sometimes be a drastic variation in fitness levels, with some students extremely fit and others very sedentary. Remember to keep an eye on energy levels of this age group, and include time for rest, making sure they are eating well and staying hydrated.

The following are some things to keep in mind when working with middle school students:

- Respect students' need for privacy.
- Emphasize the importance of school and setting goals.
- Listen without interrupting or judging.

Teaching High School Yoga: Grades 9-12

During this phase in their lives, students are trying to make sense of who they are and how they will live their adult lives, thus the period of what is called egocentrism—trying to answer the question "Who am I?" while everything revolves around them! Yoga not only is a physical activity for teens but also provides a laboratory to practice self-awareness and reflection as well as stress management—yoga is a great experience for developing both inner and outer strength in teens. It helps teens explore positive social interaction, ethical behavior, conflict resolution, and a connection to history and culture. Yoga also provides practical knowledge of the application of exercise physiology and biomechanics. For this age group, it is important to emphasize individual progress and respect for others, success toward personal goals, how what is learned in yoga connects to the outside world, and communicating trust and responsibility.

This group may challenge you by sometimes being emotionally immature; they can look and act like adults at times by showing empathy and caring, and then—boom—switch back to egocentric tendencies. This age group can also be hard to deal with when they have the "know it all" attitude, but with patience and openness and just staying with the gift of yoga, you can conquer this attitude.

These students like to do yoga that adults are doing. Mentioning examples of their favorite athletes, sports teams, or celebrities who practice yoga might motivate this age group. A variety of teaching styles works well with this group, including peer teaching.

Following are some things to keep in mind when working with high school students:

- Keep a sense of humor.
- Do not take things personally.
- Be positive in all interactions, as negativity can drag down the group's energy.

SUMMARY

Yoga is a fabulous holistic activity for students that focuses on all the aspects of healthy and balanced living including physical, spiritual, emotional, social, and global elements. Students in yoga are engaged in creative ways that allow them to enjoy movement, use their imagination, control their impulses, and learn to relax. Yoga can be a true gift we can share with our students. The next chapters provide the scientific background of the anatomical and kinesiological aspects of teaching yoga to students.

chapter

4

Scientific and Movement Principles of Yoga

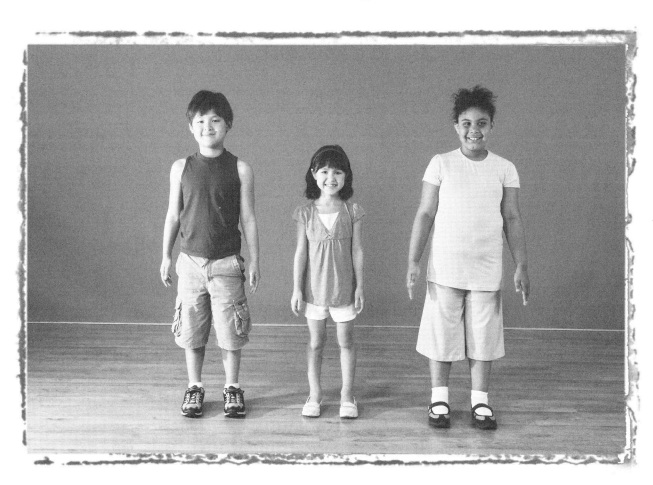

*I*n healthy and balanced living, the goal is to improve and maintain overall functional health-related fitness. Health-related fitness includes muscular strength and endurance, cardiorespiratory endurance, and flexibility. In contrast, sport-related fitness focuses on improving coordination and agility specifically linked to the sport. Yoga provides a safe environment to improve the overall health-related fitness of our students.

Understanding the movement principles is known as kinesiology, the study of human movement. Understanding these principles allows our students to improve their body awareness through improved posture, flexibility, and strength as well as learn how to relax the muscles. This chapter presents, as simply as possible, the basics of the anatomy and physiology of breathing; the role of various parts of the musculoskeletal system used for the various yoga poses; and the important scientific principles behind strength, endurance, flexibility, and relaxation. It is highly recommended that you further research the anatomy and kinesiology resources in the reference section for more-detailed explanations and information.

ANATOMY AND PHYSIOLOGY OF BREATH

Yoga teaches that the breath influences the body and mind, is the link between the body and mind, and is the foundation of yoga. Looking at babies and animals as models of correct breathing, it looks as if they use their whole bodies to breathe. Somehow as children get older, they lose this ability to breathe correctly. With our students, the task is to teach them to re-learn how to breathe, as many may use only one third to one eighth of their lung capacity. Shallow breathing, or chest breathing, cues the sympathetic nervous system to engage the fight or flight response and all the accompanying reactions, such as elevated blood pressure and heart rate. Shallow breathing contributes to fatigue and becoming cranky, which does not help students deal well with everyday life situations. In yoga, when the breath is full, it energizes the body during inhalations and gets rid of impurities during exhalations.

One of the goals of mind–body exercise is to connect with the life force, or prana energy. How we breathe has a profound effect on our levels of energy and the nervous system. Brain cells must have oxygen more than any other tissue in our bodies—in fact three times the amount. By increasing the oxygen delivered to our brains, we can strengthen what is sometimes referred to as the autonomic or automatic nervous system. The autonomic nervous system allows for breathing without conscious thought, but through mindful breathing, we can regulate the breath and thereby affect blood pressure, heart rate, the immune system, brain waves, digestion, and even sleep patterns!

In our stressful environment, we tend to fall back on habits that instinctively kept us alive when confronting threats to our existence (e.g., predators or enemies that might take our food, our offspring, or our lives). We hurl our minds and bodies into either fight or flight, which provides the body with the strength, energy, and focus to cope by fighting or running. In modern times, our lives have evolved to the point where many of us do not have these threats to our existence, but we continue to use our resources when reacting to all the stressors that pop up. Our buttons get pushed, and we are set off. The first reaction is to hyperventilate; our breath becomes choppy and shallow. While the body is springing into action, only a small part of the brain is fully utilized. This is why, when under stress, we may forget important information or think later of something we wish we had said. In yoga, we retrain ourselves to use deep and relaxing breaths to bring ourselves back to equilibrium so we can stay energized and focus on the task at hand.

Mechanics of Yoga Breath

It is evident that our students are not using their bodies to breathe correctly. Already they are slouching, and the posture muscles are becoming atrophied. It is hard to get air into the lungs if the upper body is caved in and the air is cut off. A short anatomy lesson is included here so the instruction for teaching the breath and relaxation exercises makes sense.

Two areas of the body work in concert during breathing: the thoracic cavity (or area) and the abdominal cavity (or area). The thoracic area contains the lungs and heart. The abdominal area contains the digestive organs: stomach, kidneys, liver, pancreas, bladder, and small and large intestines. During yogic breathing, the abdominal area pushes up into the thoracic area during exhalation; inversely, the thoracic area pushes down on the abdominal area during inhalation. The key muscle used in breathing is the diaphragm, located horizontally across the trunk at the bottom of the ribs below the lungs. The diaphragm separates the thoracic and abdominal cavities, and the movement of this muscle is important to the yoga breath. When relaxed, the diaphragm curves upward into the lung area. When contracted, the diaphragm pushes downward into the digestive organs, and this movement allows for the lengthening downward of the chest cavity (see figure 4.1). This makes the lung cavity bigger so the lungs can fill with more air during inhalation. As the air is expelled during exhalation, the diaphragm helps make the lung cavity smaller, therefore pushing air out of the lungs.

To take full, deep breaths, other muscles come into play as well, allowing the thoracic area to expand its capacity in two more dimensions. The intercostal muscles lie between the ribs and help the chest cavity expand outward to the sides. The muscles located at the collarbones, the sternum, the back, and the neck help expand the cavity upward. Thus, the thoracic area can expand in three directions. When we take a big breath to blow out a candle, we rely mostly on the collarbones and sternum and are often perplexed when the air is not effective. The most important area to train for increasing the breath so it is deep and relaxed is the diaphragm muscle, followed by the ribs and then the collarbones or upper chest area.

Breath and the Yoga Poses

The first goal of teaching correct breathing is to teach students to slow down their rate of breathing as well as make the breathing cycles even, thus matching the rate of inhalation to the exhalation. The second goal is to improve the vital capacity, or the strength of the breath—how much air is taken in and expelled out.

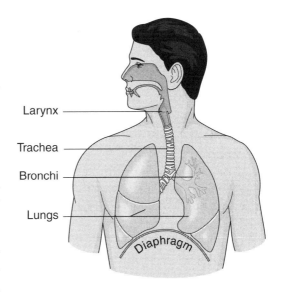

FIGURE 4.1 The anatomy of breathing.

The breath is the true teacher in yoga, as it will let the participants know if they are practicing correctly. In instructing yoga, cueing to focus and pay attention to the breath is constant. If the breath becomes awkward, jagged, or constricted, or if it becomes hard to breathe, it is crucial to back off a bit or rest until the breath can be strong again. This needs to be reinforced over and over again with cues such as "Is your breath deep and relaxed?" or "Make sure your breath starts deep in your belly and fills up your whole body during this pose."

Because yoga is a mind–body practice, sometimes emotions can bubble to the surface and make a student feel vulnerable. It may become difficult to breathe in a certain pose, and the student may feel panicky and start to hyperventilate. An example is in a back bend when the head is back and the throat opened; it may be scary for students. It is important to let the students know that this may happen while exploring poses, and if a student needs to stop the pose or just rest quietly, this is an important thing for her to do in order to deal positively with these emotions. You can also encourage a student to write about any emotions or feelings he might have had in his yoga practice that day and what he might have noticed or felt about these emotions.

Role of Breath in Stress Management

The breath has a profound effect on the nervous system. Our students come to us with numerous and varied stressors. The key aspect of stress management is our perception of the stressor. If we can teach our students to take a big breath before writing an exam or giving a speech, thus increasing the oxygen delivered to the brain and using more of the brain, the student can deal with her perception of the stressor more effectively. Also by using full diaphragmatic breath, we strengthen the parasympathetic nervous system. The parasympathetic drive of our nervous system, which can be thought of as "the rest and digest" part of the system, allows the body to deal with stressors more effectively. Using the whole brain to think through problems and to stay calm and focused when faced with challenging situations allows the body to heal and recharge itself, bringing it back to whole.

ANATOMY AND KINESIOLOGY OF THE MUSCULOSKELETAL SYSTEM

The anatomical charts provided will help you become familiar with the various muscles used in yoga (see figures 4.2 and 4.3). By becoming familiar with the muscles and muscle groups, you help students become more aware of their bodies and movement. For example, instead of saying, "Stretch your legs," your instructions can be more specific: "Engage your quadriceps while relaxing your hamstrings." In addition, using the anatomically correct terms will eliminate confusion about what is appropriate terminology for different body parts. Backside or tush might be confusing, while gluteals is very clear and direct.

The musculoskeletal system is made up of bones, joints, muscles, and connective tissue.

There are more than 600 muscles in the human body. Muscles are made up of microscopic fibers that have the ability to contract and relax, which means they can shorten and lengthen. Movement occurs when a muscle applies enough force to the bone to which it is attached, causing it to be moved or to be held in a stable position. The muscle does this by lengthening or shortening. It may be easier to

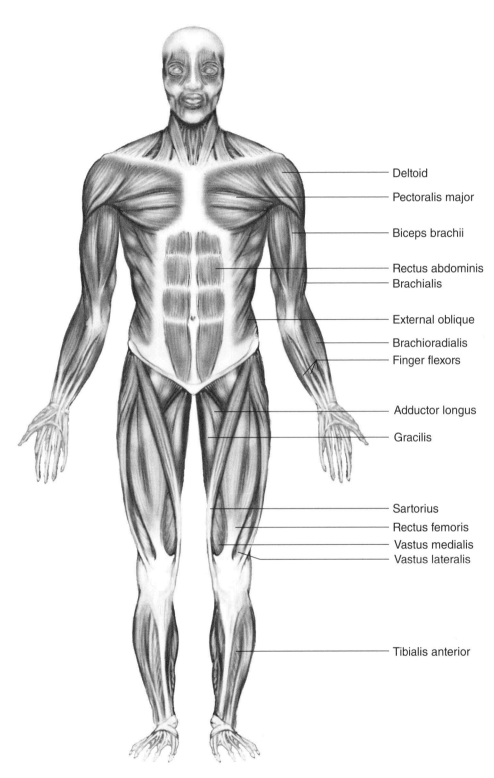

Deltoid

Pectoralis major

Biceps brachii

Rectus abdominis
Brachialis

External oblique

Brachioradialis
Finger flexors

Adductor longus

Gracilis

Sartorius
Rectus femoris
Vastus medialis
Vastus lateralis

Tibialis anterior

FIGURE 4.2 Anterior view.

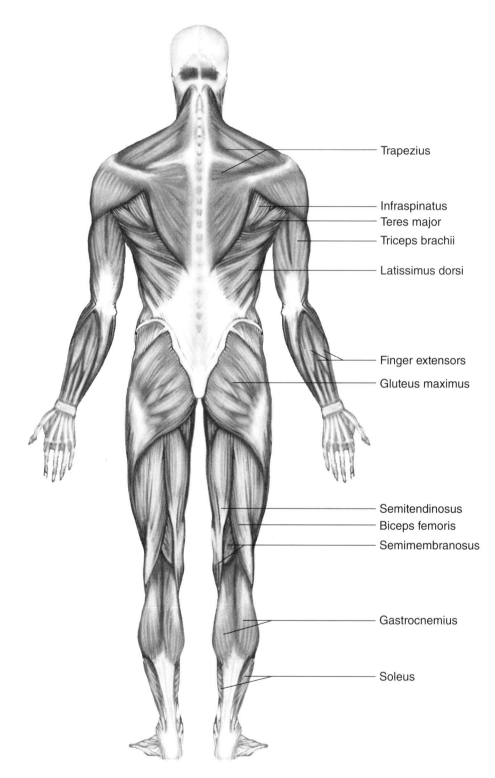

Trapezius

Infraspinatus
Teres major
Triceps brachii

Latissimus dorsi

Finger extensors
Gluteus maximus

Semitendinosus
Biceps femoris
Semimembranosus

Gastrocnemius

Soleus

FIGURE 4.3 Posterior view.

understand that muscles work in pairs and act in opposition to create movement. Typically when one muscle lengthens, the other muscle in the pair or group contracts, or shortens. An example is, as a glass of water is brought to the mouth, the biceps contracts and the triceps lengthens.

Depending on the movement, muscles take on specific roles. For example, when the upper arm is moved away from the side of the body (e.g., raising the arm away from the side of the body to overhead), the deltoid (the muscles on top of the shoulder joint) is known as the prime mover. The deltoid is contracting, and nearby muscles known as synergists contract and assist to hold the shoulder stable. Other muscles act as antagonists. These muscles resist the prime mover's action. If both the prime mover and antagonist contract at the same time, there will be rigid movement. Muscles work together with each other to create smooth, coordinated movement.

In yoga, the goal is a healthy balance of strength and flexibility. Each pose is a dynamic blend of strength and stretch and provides what we see as "muscle tone" (i.e., the muscles are strong and able to move easily around the joints). What can happen when asking students to relax is the muscle may actually be in contraction, making it impossible to relax. To help students better stretch the muscle, it is helpful to cue them to relax into the stretch. If a muscle is moved suddenly, the muscle actually responds by reflexively shortening to protect itself from injury, which is the exact opposite of what is intended.

SCIENCE OF FLEXIBILITY

Understanding how the body best responds to stretching and thus improving flexibility is important when teaching yoga. It is amazing to continue to see professional athletes using unsound stretching principles (and coaches allowing their athletes to use them), such as forcing the muscle beyond its stretch, using ballistic or bouncing movements while stretching, or putting the joints in positions that hurt or injure the joint.

Range of Motion

The range of motion is the ability of the muscles surrounding a specific joint to move freely; it is joint specific. For example, the hip joint has less of a range of motion than the shoulder joint. Part of this ability to move freely can be increased through improving the flexibility of the muscles attached to the joint. Muscles are able to stretch and return to their original shape. In fact, they can stretch up to 170% without damage. What limits flexibility is the connective tissue involved. Connective tissue is made up of noncontractile (nonmoving) cells that are tough, are fibrous, and vary in flexibility. Connective tissue includes cartilage, ligaments, tendons, and fascia.

Cartilage is a tough, elastic-like connective tissue. It covers the ends of bones at the joints and is found at the ends of the ribs, between the symphysis pubis, and in the nose and ears. Cartilage provides a limited amount of flexibility. Ligaments are tough, fibrous bands that connect bone to bone (e.g., the ligaments connecting the bones of the knee). Anyone who has torn knee ligaments knows that these tissues unfortunately do not regenerate like bones or muscles and have very limited flexibility. The tendons are bands of tissue that connect muscle to bone (e.g., the Achilles tendon that attaches the heel bone to the calf muscle). Similar to ligaments, tendons have limited flexibility, and overstretching

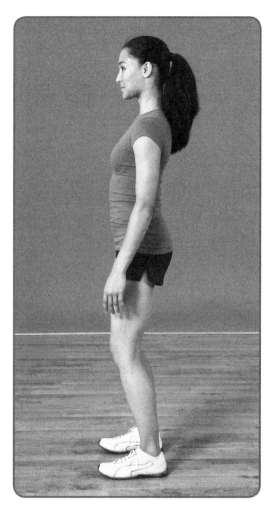

FIGURE 4.4 Correct knee alignment.

tendons or ligaments is discouraged. A common example of overstretching is hyperextending the knee joint by locking the joint when doing a forward fold, either standing or sitting. It is recommended to slightly bend the knees, to keep them "soft" in order to protect the joint and safely stretch the hamstring muscle group (muscles at the back of the upper leg) (see figure 4.4).

Stretch Reflex

The principle that allows a muscle to be stretched but not overstretched, causing injury, is called the stretch reflex. Within the muscles are sensory receptors called muscle spindles, which are specialized muscle fibers. Muscle spindles are one of the proprioceptors, specialized sensory receptors that are sensitive to stretch, tension, and pressure within the muscles, joints, and tendons and provide information on the tension of the muscle fibers. The muscle as well as the ligaments and tendons associated with it are protected from overstretching and injury by these muscle spindles. These organs quickly relay information to both the conscious and unconscious parts of the nervous system. When a muscle is placed in excessive stretch or under ballistic or bouncing movement, the muscle spindles and muscle fibers are signaled by the nervous system to protect themselves and shorten.

The static stretch, or the held stretch that is practiced in yoga, is optimized by moving slowly into the pose and holding it for sustained periods of time, thus optimizing the stretch and flexibility. When holding a stretch, yoga participants initially notice a bit of resistance from the protective reaction of the muscle spindles, but with a sustained stretch, a secondary reaction allows the fibers to slowly lengthen. As the muscle moves toward its optimal length, the sensation felt is a restricting tightness followed by warmth in the area, allowing for the stretch to be explored further or deeper. If the sensation is burning or a spasm, this input is clearly saying "time to back off." Paying attention to input from the body can help students differentiate and become aware of the correct amount of stretch.

Teaching our students how to stretch correctly and maintain flexibility is important for healthy and balanced living by providing ease of everyday movement, improved posture, and improved balance. Next we'll look at more of the numerous benefits of flexibility.

Benefits of Stretching

One of the benefits of yoga is the improvement of our students' flexibility. There are numerous benefits of remaining flexible throughout the life span:

- Competency in other physical activities
- Functional independence in activities of daily living
- Ability to maintain range of motion of joints and surrounding tissue
- Improved posture and decreased lower-back problems
- Decreased muscle soreness, aches, and overall pain
- Injury prevention

Many of the benefits derived from stretching, such as improved joint lubrication, healing, circulation, and range of motion, are brought about by changing the flexibility of the fascia. The fascia are dense, weblike tissues that surround, intertwine, and weave into the muscles and organs, holding them in place and separating them. The flexibility of the fascia surrounding the muscle can be improved over time. In theory, when a muscle fiber is stretched, it can elongate up to 170% of its resting length. What comes into the mix is the fascia covering the muscle and interwoven into the muscle fibers. Fascia can through inactivity become rigid and less able to stretch, but with consistent and correct stretching it can remain flexible and allow the muscles to stay flexible as well. To do this, the science of stretching suggests holding the stretch for 90 to 120 seconds. Yoga primarily uses static stretching; this means the stretch is held without movement. Many benefits can be gained by holding a slow, comfortable stretch; keeping the breath full and relaxed; and slowly relaxing into the stretch as well as slowly coming out of the stretch. Keep in mind that after an injury, the resulting scar tissue is made up of collagen, which is not flexible and may limit the range of motion.

Flexibility is influenced by several other factors such as body temperature, hydration, and breath. The body's core temperature should be elevated so the muscles can relax better. Having the room temperature comfortably warm and encouraging students to hydrate can enhance this process. Relaxed breathing allows the parasympathetic nervous system to take over and promote relaxation.

BUILDING A HEALTHY AND STRONG SPINE

The foundation of human movement comes from the spine. The musculature of the spine requires a balance of both flexibility and the strength that yoga provides. This balance includes proper contraction and relaxation of opposing muscles. A strong and healthy spine is important for the holistic health of our students.

One of the most common complaints among adults is back pain, which can be caused by a number of reasons, mainly inactivity, obesity, and faulty lifting mechanics. Unfortunately, many of our students already exhibit unhealthy spinal postures that influence their energy, emotions, ability to learn, and self-esteem. Sadly, our students may also be vulnerable to back pain because they are spending less time being active, are heavier, and do not have strong core (trunk) muscles to support the back. Starting early on back health is important. A brief explanation of the anatomy and kinesiology of the spine is presented to give you an understanding of the mechanics of the spine and posture.

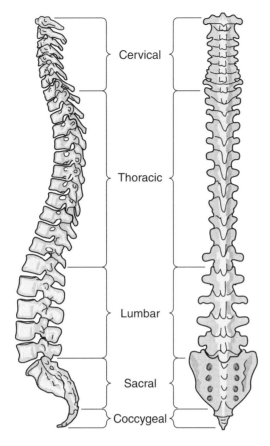

FIGURE 4.5 The bones of the spinal column.

The bones of the spine are called vertebrae (see figure 4.5). The size and shape of the vertebrae vary depending on their function and placement in the spinal column. The neck vertebrae are smaller than the thick lumbar (lower back) vertebrae that need to be hefty so the large muscles of the back can attach to them. The spine can be visualized as a string of beads—bigger beads at the bottom gradually becoming smaller. The big beads or vertebrae have discs (intervertebral discs) between them. These discs have fluid in them similar to jelly in a jelly doughnut, and the discs protect the vertebrae and serve as shock absorbers. As the body ages, the cushioning provided by the discs slowly deteriorates, mostly because of inactivity. Most back problems originate in the discs in the lumbar area, but the supporting features of this area also come into play, including ligaments, facet joints, intervertebral discs, and musculature of the spine. Through correct movement, the spine can be kept flexible and supple by allowing the discs to be nourished, as they do not have their own blood supply but derive nutrients from the vertebral end plates.

Starting at the base of the spine, the coccyx (or tailbone) is made up of 4 bones that are fused together. The lower back consists of the sacrum, which is 5 sacral vertebrae that are fused into one bone, and the 5 lumbar vertebrae. Next are the 12 thoracic vertebrae that make up the upper part of the spine and finally the 7 cervical vertebrae that make up the neck area. There are four natural spinal curves at the cervical, thoracic, lumbar, and coccygeal/sacral areas.

The spine has primary and secondary curves. The primary curves are the thoracic and sacral curves. When an infant starts her development from birth, the primary curves are developed. The primary curve at the cervical and thoracic area is developed when the infant begins to lift her head, then sits up, followed by creeping and crawling, allowing the growing child to support the weight of her head. The secondary curve of the lumbar area is developed as the child begins to stand, bear weight, and later walk. The curves give support and are designed to provide shock absorption.

The spine can move in four different ways. The basic spinal movements are flexion, as in a forward fold; extension, as seen in mountain pose; side to side (also called lateral flexion), as in quarter moon pose; and rotation, or twisting right to left, as in twisted chair pose (see figure 4.6).

Another factor that affects spine alignment is the strength of the core muscles. The core muscles are important for lower-back strength and function, thereby influencing tasks of everyday living such as moving the body and lifting objects.

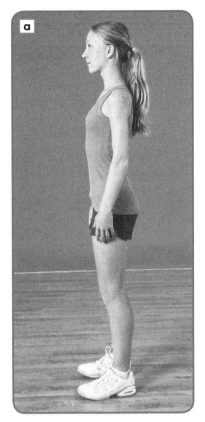

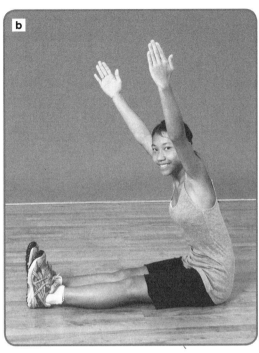

FIGURE 4.6 (a) A healthy posture, (b) spinal flexion, (c) spinal extension, (d) lateral flexion of the spine, and (e) rotation of the spine.

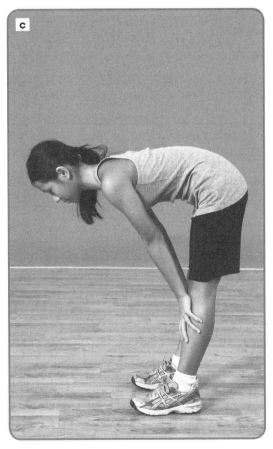

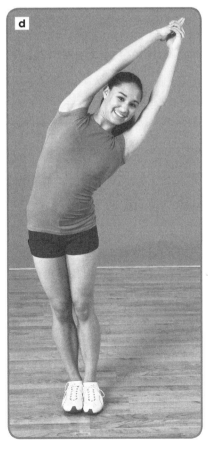

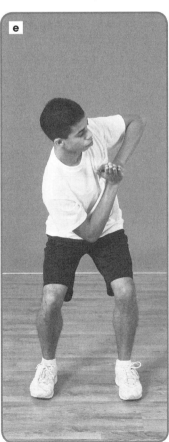

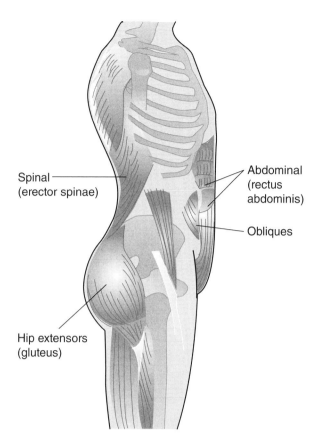

Spinal
(erector spinae)

Abdominal
(rectus
abdominis)

Obliques

Hip extensors
(gluteus)

FIGURE 4.7 The core muscles.

Core Muscles

Yoga poses are practiced with a focus on the fundamental muscles that help maintain the integrity of the spine. These muscles are called the core muscles. The core muscles include the rectus abdominis muscles that run vertically from the pubic bone to the sternum and the transverse abdominis muscle, which runs like a seat belt horizontally across the hip area. The oblique muscles are also included in the core group; they attach the hip and the ribs, define the waist, and allow for twisting movements (see figure 4.7). Traditional "abs of steel" exercise programs often emphasize only the front of the body and not the entire core, which includes the muscles of the upper and lower back and the gluteal area that also help maintain the strength of the core. Much of human movement moves from the core outward. For instance, when lifting a heavy box safely, the core muscles are emphasized and not just the legs.

Posture

Yoga emphasizes the importance of correct posture in order to maintain a strong spine and ease of spinal movement. Correct posture also affects breathing, movement efficiency, and energy. In chapter 3, developing and improving students' posture is identified as an important developmental milestone. Yoga is an excellent tool for improving posture.

Posture influences students' body concept, energy, and emotional states. For example, when the body starts to slump (e.g., slouching by rounding the shoulders, caving in the chest and heart space, stressing the cervical vertebrae as the head droops forward), the body becomes fatigued as its ability to receive oxygen is diminished in this closed-off posture.

Starting with younger students, it is important for them to understand good posture mechanics. This can be emphasized in how they sit at their desks doing work or at their computers. Students can be made aware of how they walk and carry books or backpacks that can be extremely heavy and cause injury. Teaching correct lifting mechanics is also important for younger students.

Often in adolescence when there are growth spurts, a student may be much taller than his peers, or during puberty a female student may be more developed in the bust area. These students may slouch to hide their bodies. The postural muscles become weak and atrophied, making it even harder for the students to stand and sit up straight. Needless to say, posture is important for lifelong health. You can help develop your students' awareness of good posture by pointing out good upper-body posture. This can be done not only in yoga class but also whenever students are doing any movement, sitting or standing.

The bones and the primary muscles of posture include the following (see figures 4.2 and 4.3 on pages 51 and 52):

- Clavicles (collarbones): pectorals
- Spine: erector spinae
- Scapulae (shoulder blades): trapezius, latissimus dorsi, rhomboids

In yoga, function is more important than form. This means the body is never compromised for the sake of achieving a certain pose. This requires teaching correct spinal alignment in order for the spine to remain healthy and functional. The importance of being mindful of the body and moving correctly while respecting individual needs and limitations must be reinforced over and over. Cues such as "Check into your body to make sure it feels right" and "Yoga should feel good!" may help bolster this vital concept.

TEACHING YOGA POSES

For the purpose of instruction, we present the general poses followed by suggestions for modifying the poses, referred to as variations for different age groups and abilities. These suggested age groups are in general; as you know, a 5-year-old can be as developmentally advanced as a 7- or 8-year-old, who can be in the same class with a student lagging behind in development. In addition, some students may be physically able to do more-advanced poses but emotionally have problems concentrating or listening to directions.

Infusion ideas are included with the poses. Infusion ideas are ways to enrich the learning experience by infusing other topics and subjects into the yoga class, making it a holistic activity. The instructions provided are as simple as possible, with a beginning stance or posture and a finishing stance or posture. Often, the finishing pose suggested is considered a balancing pose. In this case, balancing means bringing balance to the whole body. For example, if the pose involves a back bend or the spine is extended, then the finishing pose would involve back flexion to allow for a balanced practice.

Your role as an instructor is to help the students take responsibility for their own self-care, meaning they find the best way to do the pose or find a pose that works for them. This can be thought of as "fake it until you make it." For example, in a balancing pose, encourage students to use a prop such as a wall or chair to help them balance so they don't become frustrated and give up because they are not able to do the pose as presented.

To stay consistent and to avoid confusion, the names included are the traditional Western translations of the Sanskrit names for the poses. Also provided after each traditional name are alternative names meant to sound like fun and be more accessible. Feel free to adapt the names to fit your teaching because many of the names of poses are just made up.

Five Steps for Introducing a Yoga Pose

How you introduce a yoga pose will always depend on the age and developmental level of the students, but here are some general suggestions.

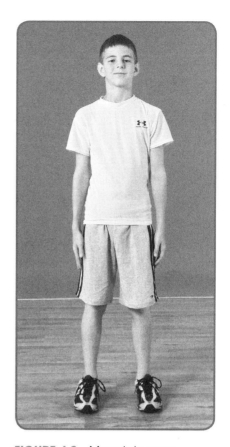

FIGURE 4.8　Mountain pose.

- Before starting instructing a pose, ask all students to be quiet and still for a few breaths. You can make a few comments about the intention of the pose or tell a story connected to the pose.

- Set the tone by giving direction for the breath. Some cues to facilitate this include "Listen to your breath as if you are listening to the sound coming from a sea shell," or "Listen quietly to your breath as you breathe in and out through your heart."

- Make sure that breath is linked with the pose. For example, for mountain pose you might say, "Take a big breath in, and at the same time lift your heart and let your arms reach up to the sky and tickle the clouds" (see figure 4.8). Think of yoga as a dance of movements that are connected to the rhythm of the breath. Typically, on inhalation, the body is moved in order to be open to receive oxygen; on exhalation, the body is moved to release toxins and carbon dioxide.

- Bring students' awareness to the energy or the intention of the pose. For example, for tree pose you might say, "The supporting or balancing leg is like a strong tree trunk, with the foot growing strong roots deep in the ground below." Back bends provide another example. When the spine bends backward, the area around the heart opens up. Ask the students when they practice this pose to keep the area around the heart open and find the middle ground, that balance between effort and challenge mixed with comfort and ease.

- Before starting a pose or a movement, it is important to feel grounded and centered, to have a foundation. In yoga, the body needs to be strongly grounded at all times. The feet are the foundation when standing, and the sit bones (the ischium bones) are the foundation when sitting. Similar to building a house, where the foundation allows for floors to be build on top of it, a strong foundation allows the rest of the body to be correctly and safely aligned.

Step-by-Step Teaching of Correct Alignment

Equally important in setting the tone and foundation for each yoga pose is alignment.

Alignment refers to the stature of the body that allows for optimal body mechanics and posture. It is important to note that the alignment principles are not lost or forgotten when the body starts to move. Whether the pose is mountain or seated forward fold with the legs straight out in front, correct alignment still applies (see figure 4.9). Even in final relaxation posture, the body should feel lengthened and open.

The best example to illustrate the concept of feeling grounded, centered, and in alignment is mountain pose, which is the standing pose from which all standing poses begin. If you imagine a mountain, the base is strongly rooted into the ground while the peaks aspire into the clouds and the sky. The following steps describe alignment using mountain pose as the reference. It is easy to see how mountain pose is named, with the analogous lower body firmly grounded, the spine strong, and the heart and upper body open and lifted.

1. Spread the toes wide, making floor contact with all four parts of the foot: the ball of the foot, pinky toe side, and inner and outer heel. The feet are hip-width apart, with the feet firmly placed into the floor. Briefly lift the toes to allow for the body weight to be shifted back. Then release the toes, and be mindful not to grip with the toes.

2. Actively engage the muscles of the legs, with the knees slightly bent. "Actively" engaging muscles means contracting and making the muscles firm in the area. Engage the abdomen, or core, of the body as if putting on a seat belt, keeping the area from the hips to the shoulders (core) strong and stable but not rigid. The tailbone will naturally tuck down and under to point to the floor, which helps stabilize the back muscles.

3. Stand tall, finding length through the spine with the crown of the head reaching toward the sky. Honor the natural curves of the spine, and keep the head as a natural extension of the spine, not hyperextended or arched back. Imagine a string with a weight attached to it and hanging from the ceiling next to you. This string will bisect the ears, shoulders, hips, knees, and ankles.

4. From the belly button down, there is a strong foundation. With the feet rooted into the ground, the legs are strong as if the muscles are squeezing the bones, and the kneecaps are slightly lifted, with the muscles of the quadriceps (front of the upper legs) engaged.

5. From the belly button up, the upper body is open and lifted out of the waist but not rigid. Place the head at the top of the spine, the chin level with the ground. Keep the chest open and lift the heart space, the collarbones wide. Roll the shoulder blades back and down as if they are reaching to the back pockets. Do not let the shoulders hunch, creating a lot of space between the ears and shoulders.

Take a look at the elements of alignment shown in the two alignment examples of mountain pose (see figures 4.8 and 4.9).

Holding of Poses

The holding of a yoga pose refers to how long the pose is held or maintained in order for the benefits of the pose, such as muscle endurance, strength, or flexibility, to be realized. To

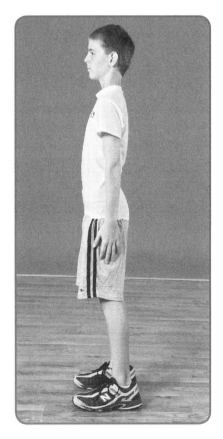

FIGURE 4.9 Side view of the mountain pose.

improve these areas, the principle of overload must be applied. One way of looking at overload is finding the middle path, or the edge. To gain strength, endurance, or flexibility, we must challenge the body in order for growth to occur, but not to a point where there is discomfort or pain. This can be facilitated by asking students to stay with the pose so they feel challenged but not overdoing it and becoming frustrated. You need to continually point out that yoga should feel good. Your language to students must include "permission language," which is discussed in chapter 3. This means giving students the responsibility of being the best judge of what their bodies need, what their middle path is, and when to come out of a pose. Ways to encourage this permission is to state during a pose, "You can hold this pose for one or two breaths and then come in and out of the pose when you need to."

Yoga poses should have a natural ebb and flow to them. This means an intention of a moderate level of steady and comfortable effort and not a goal to push to exhaustion and then collapse. With younger students, it is important to pace the more-active poses with restful poses, going back and forth between play and rest. Paying close attention to your students' breathing and energy levels can cue you as to what is the right mix for them. With older students, encourage the importance of mixing up the effort and rest. An example of an activity that promotes rest is Take Five.

TAKE FIVE

Lying prone (on the belly), arms folded in front with the head resting on the hands, use the next five (take five) exhalations to focus on relaxing a different part of the body, and allow yourself to relax and melt down into the floor. Cue the students as follows:

1. "Exhale 1, and let your legs melt into the floor."
2. "Exhale 2, and let your arms become heavy and warm."
3. "Exhale 3, and soften the belly."
4. "Exhale 4, and let the heart space be peaceful."
5. "Exhale 5, and let the whole body melt down into the floor."

Nonrecommended Poses

Although most yoga poses are safer than many common sports and activities students participate in, some poses are not appropriate for young children and are not included in this book. This is not necessarily a matter of difficulty but rather the effect on their growing bodies. These include headstand, fish pose, hero pose, and shoulder stand. Handstands are also not included; they may be suitable for small groups but are not recommended for general classes. However, there are many poses that are simple and can be included in a safe and fun program. Keep in mind that the art of teaching any subject is adapting for each person; if a pose doesn't feel right for a particular group or your comfort zone as an instructor, honor that opinion and do not include it.

SUMMARY

Using instruction that emphasizes each student's unique anatomy and physiology needs to be constantly reinforced. A cue to help emphasize each student's individuality is "Everyone's body is different; you need to concentrate on your own stretch and never compete." Students may think that forcing or bouncing may illicit a deeper stretch. However, cueing the students to find their edge, meaning finding that point in the stretch where they feel sensation but not pushing beyond that, as if slowly stretching a rubber band, will help students find their optimal stretch.

Now that the students know the principles of yoga, how to breathe, and how to move correctly in yoga, introducing the poses and exercises allows the students to apply these important lessons to creative and fun movement.

chapter

5

Yoga Lesson and Unit Plans

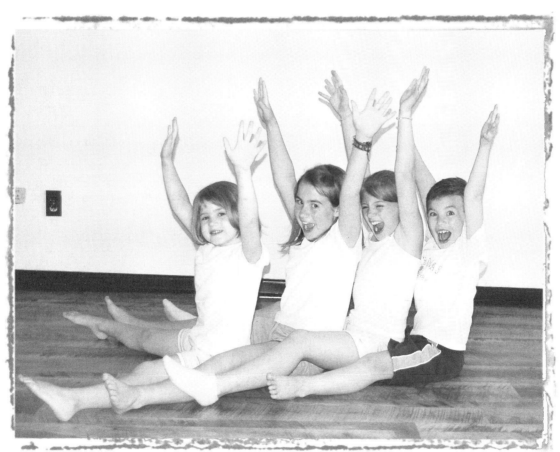

Yoga is an exceptional activity for educating the whole child. With this intention, the yoga lesson plan should be designed to allow for flow and maximum participation and benefits for all students. A yoga lesson can follow a traditional fitness workout with a warm-up, activity phase, and cool-down. This model lets the students settle into their breath and focus on the yoga session, then slowly progress into the cardiorespiratory and strength-enhancing sequence of poses, and finally reap the benefits of the physical practice of the yoga asanas by allowing the body and mind to relax and rejuvenate. This does not mean this model needs to be strictly adhered to; use it as a general guideline of starting in a breath-focused centering phase, moving into an active phase that can be mixed with restful poses, and finishing with a relaxation phase and closing ritual.

This chapter covers the pragmatic aspects of planning for yoga classes. This includes how to sequence and allot time for the various segments of the class such as the opening, the workout, and relaxation times. Sample lesson plans are offered for various age groups and groups of students (e.g., athletes) to provide an idea of how to creatively design classes. An example of a unit plan is included to suggest a way to introduce yoga poses over the course of a time period such as a weekly class at a yoga studio or recreation center for children or a week-long yoga unit in a physical education curriculum. The suggestions offered are general, and different circumstances will require adaptations.

YOGA LESSON PLAN

The outline provided in table 5.1 can help start the creative juices flowing in planning yoga experiences for your students. The table provides a general idea of the time allotment for the various age groups. As stated in the introduction to this chapter, this outline offers a sequence that is well established in the physical education field. For example, the lesson plan is set up to present poses that are best practiced with the body warmed up toward the middle to end of the session.

There is always time for yoga. Whether this means taking only 1 minute to relax the breath, using 3 minutes to relax the body from head to toe while the students are lying down or in a chair, or sharing a 30-minute yoga class with your students, it is all good and beneficial. One of the most profound aspects of yoga is how quickly the benefits of having a relaxed state of mind or feeling energized can be realized within a short period of time. In the classroom or gym, the students' energy will change very quickly for the better by using the tools learned in yoga.

With preschool students, a yoga class is best limited to 30 minutes or less, while a teen class can last up to 60 minutes. Most yoga classes for adults allow teens to sign up, but these classes typically last 75 minutes, and from experience that becomes a little too long for teens. The time allotments for the warm-up, workout (or active) phase, and closing are guidelines only. Pay close attention to the students' ability to focus, their energy level, their body language, their enthusiasm, the noise level, and the temperature of the room, and adjust the time accordingly.

Lesson Plan Outline

The lesson plan outline provided here is an example of a method to plan and reflect on the yoga classes for your students.

TABLE 5.1 Time Allotment for Yoga Class

	Warm-up	Workout	Closing
Preschool/ages 3-5 (15-30 min)	Breathing exercises and sharing time 5-10 min	Games and movement activities 5-10 min	Relaxing stretches and story time 5-10 min
Lower elementary/ages 5-7 (25-45 min)	Warm-up poses, breathing exercises, and sharing time 5-10 min	Games, movement activities, and standing and balancing poses 15-20 min	Floor poses and relaxation time 10-15 min
Upper elementary/ages 8-12 (25-45 min)	Warm-up poses and breathing exercises 5-10 min	Standing and balancing poses, sun salutation, cooperative games, and partner poses 15-20 min	Floor poses, relaxation time, and discussion time 5-15 min
High school/ages 13-17 (45-60 min)	Breathing exercises, meditation exercises, and seated poses 10-15 min	Flowing yoga sequences interspersed with standing and balancing poses; partner poses 20-25 min	Core poses on floor, deep stretch and relaxation time, discussion and reflection time, and closing meditation 15-20 min

1. **Date of lesson, group, amount of time, setting.**

2. **Purpose or theme of the lesson:** What will the students learn in this lesson? It might be linked to the last lesson or an end-of-lesson objective. For example, students did the tree pose alone last class, and now they will cooperate with other students to make a forest of trees, or the class is learning to link several poses from past classes into a flowing sequence. An example of a theme might be a heart-focused yoga class where healthy heart content is infused within the yoga class. More ideas on infusion are found in the next chapter.

3. **Physical education standard addressed:** See the NASPE standards on page 6.

4. **Teacher objective:** What is your objective for improving your teaching?

5. **Yoga space:** This includes a diagram and description of where students and equipment (if needed) are going to be. Planning ahead for this is important. For example, you might need an electrical outlet for music, but the students are set up in a space where there is no outlet or no one can hear the music. Make sure the yoga space is safe and clean. You may need to plan extra time to set up the space, such as moving chairs or any obstacles that might interfere with the students' movement, taking a dry mop to the floor, warming up the room, or getting out mats or blankets. If you are lucky to have a designated space to use every class, it is nice to have the room all set up before the students arrive, with perhaps some music playing and the lights lowered if possible. Have an assistant to help you if there is a rush setting up the room so that when the students arrive, you are centered and relaxed and ready to share yoga.

6. **Equipment needed for this lesson:** Make sure you have enough equipment for maximum participation. Students can also share equipment or set up stations with equipment.

7. **Planned lesson activities:**

   a. Introductory or opening exercise: poem, breath, quiet reading, music

   b. Warm-up

   c. Workout: activities, standing poses, balancing poses, sequenced poses, games, and so on

   d. Floor exercises and cool-down

   e. Relaxation

   f. Closing

8. **Brief reflection:** Assess how well you met your student and teacher objectives.

Planning your lessons and then having time to reflect on them will help enrich both your yoga experience and that of your students. The lesson plan is not a rigid plan but a guide for your class instruction. Keeping the plan on an index card or on a piece of paper tucked inside a plastic sleeve to look at during class will help keep the class on track. Filing the cards or lesson plans with reflective notes will give you a ready reference for future classes.

Just a comment on the reflection part of the lesson plan. People may react to the word *assessment* as being synonymous with testing. However, assessment here is not to assign a grade but to objectively evaluate how the class went in relation to the learning objectives. Reflection is intended to answer the following questions: "What did I want to teach and have the students experience versus what actually happened?" "What can I do better next time?" Teaching is an art, and the intention of reflection is to explore experiences and insights so each class is a step along a wonderful path of teaching and living yoga.

Checklist for Planning a Yoga Lesson

One way to both plan and reflect on your teaching is to use a checklist to guide your choice of poses, exercises, games, and so on for your classes. This checklist can help you quickly judge whether what you have chosen will provide the best yoga experiences:

- Does the activity provide for differences in the skill levels of your students (i.e., is it developmentally and instructionally appropriate)?
- Can all students be successful and, at the same time, challenged?
- Does the activity provide for maximum participation and practice time?
- Can you assess if you met the student learning and teaching objectives?

The checklist is a way to keep the lesson and the instructor focused on what is good teaching for the students, but as mentioned in chapter 3, it is important to keep an open mind and heart when teaching yoga. This means that planning is important, but going with the flow of the energy and needs of the students is the key to a successful yoga plan.

SAMPLE LESSON PLANS

In this section, there are several examples of lesson plans that can be modified for a variety of settings. A classroom setting for kindergarten could be modified for a preschool facility; a physical education class in a gymnasium space could be modified for an after-school program setting; an indoor activity at a summer camp setting could be modified for a classroom or middle school field day experience; and a lesson plan for teens taking a class at a yoga studio could be modified for an athletic team's indoor practice.

Sample Lesson Plan for Preschool Students

The sample lesson plan for preschool students fuses two things this age group loves: movement and stories. The example here includes poses with a nautical theme to link with a story that might have a theme of visiting an island or going on a boat ride. The instructor can show everyone the pictures from the story. The pictures can be enlarged and laminated or put into plastic sleeves or displayed on the walls of the classroom for students to look at as they do the poses. It is fun and creative to make up different names for the poses to mimic the theme or characters of the book. For example, tree pose can be a lighthouse to connect to the nautical-themed lesson.

Date of lesson, group, amount of time, setting
Preschool students, 30-minute class, after lunch in classroom in activity space. With preschool it is recommended that there be a 1:7 ratio of adults or helpers (this could be older students) to students.

Purpose or theme of the lesson
Introduction to rules of practicing yoga in the classroom, basic yoga poses, and infusion of a story. The story in this example might be a visit to an island or going for a boat ride.

Physical education standard addressed
Standard 5: Exhibits responsible personal and social behavior that respects self and others in physical activity settings.

Teacher objective
This is the first class to introduce yoga as a special activity after lunch. The objective is to remain open and enjoy bringing yoga to the students while establishing Standard 5.

Yoga space
Move chairs and desk to open up activity space so students have room to move but understand boundaries of space.

Equipment needed for this lesson
Activity mat (carpet squares) for each student, large piece of newsprint, tape, marker, Beanie Babies, music, and storybook.

Introductory or opening exercise
Students suggest rules for sharing the activity space and for yoga, with instructor guidance. The rules are listed on a large piece of paper to color in later in the day and keep in the activity space for further reference and review. (5 minutes)

Warm-up
Seated balloon breath. Table pose and then moving in and out of cat and cow poses. Child pose. (3 minutes)

Workout
Sun salute dance. The sequence of poses that are linked together in the sun salute dance are as follows:

1. Mountain. Reach for the sky. Forward dive and hug the knees. Come to the floor onto the tummy.
2. Cobra.
3. Downward-facing dog.
4. Jump forward to hands, and unfold by doing a reverse forward dive or rolling the spine up slowly back to mountain.

Different variations of the sun salute dance include mixing in various poses such as tree or warrior. Music can be played and when it stops, it is a signal to the students to freeze into a designated pose or their favorite pose. (7 minutes)

Floor exercises and cool-down
Boat pose. Shark pose. Swimming pose. (Use any floor and cooling-down poses that follow the characters or theme of the story that will be read aloud during relaxation. (3 minutes)

Relaxation
All the students have a Beanie Baby on their bellies, and they use balloon breath to make the Beanie Babies swim up and down. (3 minutes)

Closing
Reading of story while students are in a relaxation pose. Seated in a circle: How does yoga make you feel? (infusing by reviewing importance of rules) (9 minutes)

Brief reflection
How did the students follow the rules during this new activity? How did you feel about the flow of the class and the energy level? How could other books be infused into the lesson?

Sample Lesson Plan for Grades K-2

The sample lesson plan for elementary students is ideal for an open space that allows students to move (e.g., a space the size of half a gymnasium or half a basketball court). If you have only an activity space where desk and chairs need to be moved, that is fine, just make sure to remove any obstacles and use sticky mats (described in chapter 3) so there is a nonskid surface.

Date of lesson, group, amount of time, setting
Grade 2 students, 30-minute class, in the gymnasium.

Purpose or theme of the lesson
This is a physical education class with the goal of students learning different movement patterns as well as mixing in various yoga poses.

Physical education standard addressed
Standard 2: Demonstrates understanding of movement concepts, principles, strategies, and tactics as they apply to the learning and performance of physical activities.

Teacher objective
Incorporating yoga poses within a more-traditional physical education class.

Yoga space
Half of gymnasium space with curtains between other classes. It is difficult to hear music and to regulate the lights or noise level in this kind of space for yoga. Students will be on mats in a circle.

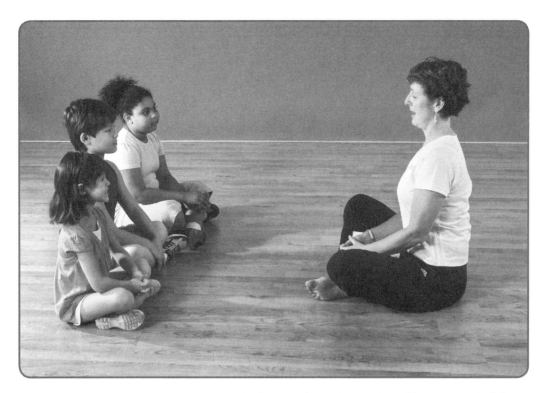

Be sure to close lessons by talking about what has been learned and how students felt about the activities.

Equipment needed for this lesson
Yoga mat for each student.

Introductory or opening exercise
Balloon breath. Bunny breath. Remind students that it is important to breathe during the exercises. (3 minutes)

Warm-up
Ask students to explore and discover different ways they can walk: pigeon (toes pointed in), duck (toes pointed outward), slide sideways, backward, on the toes and heels, bend one knee up, stick (stiff) legs, wiggle, hop ("Wiggle your nose like a bunny"). (5 minutes)

Workout
1. Standing on individual mats.
   ▪ Sun and moon salute: Prepare the students by saying, "Stand and get really tall so we can reach the clouds!" Do mountain, touch the clouds and the sun (reach up overhead), forward dive, and slowly let the sun set. Tell students to sit in their rocket chairs (chair pose). Now lift off and reach back to the sun with arms overhead, fingers laced and index fingers together, and do quarter moon poses right and left. Repeat. (2 minutes)
   ▪ Do warrior I, warrior II, and warrior III. (2 minutes)
2. On the floor. Students will sit on their own mats, will stand, and will move around the room.

▦ Cue students: "Let's go to a jungle! First we need to get into our boats [boat]. Look, we can see a crocodile [crocodile], and there's a snake [cobra]. Oh, look up, there is a monkey [the students move the way a monkey does], elephant [elephant], giraffe [students move the way a giraffe does]. OK, jump back into your boat and row really hard back [boat with rowing arms]—the crocodiles are chasing us!" (3 minutes)

3. Standing. Balancing poses back in a circle on individual mats.

▦ Pretend you are in the park. Imagine you are seeing trees (tree), birds in the trees (eagle), and statues (standing bow). (3 minutes)

Floor exercises and cool-down
Everyone walks slowly around the room. Pretend you have a slow-motion camera. Tell your students to watch you and, when you put up your hand, to stop and do one of the new poses they learned today on any mat. (2 minutes)

Relaxation
Students lying down on individual mats do starfish relaxation. (5 minutes)

Closing
Ask your students, "Today we learned different ways we can move and some fun poses. What did you like about today? Let's finish our class today with balloon breaths. Let's do 5 all together." (5 minutes)

Brief reflection
How did the students enjoy yoga as a physical education activity? How was teaching yoga different from traditional physical education activities for this age group? How did you feel about the flow of the class and the energy level?

Sample Lesson Plan for Grades 6-8

The sample lesson plan for middle school, or grades 6-8, is for a summer camp indoor activity. The activities are designed to help this particular age group work on cooperation and communication. Often this age group can be unmercifully cruel to each other, with a lot of bickering, picking on each other, and isolating members of the group. The activities provided for this age group are suggested because there is not much of the needed practice and modeling of working together, active listening, and being respectful to each other in the rest of their life experiences.

Date of lesson, group, amount of time, setting
Group of 12 campers for 45 minutes on a rainy afternoon in a carpeted activity space during quiet or siesta time.

Purpose or theme of the lesson
Cooperation—this group will be doing future camp activities that require them to work together.

Physical education standard addressed
Standard 6: Values physical activity for health, enjoyment, challenge, self-expression, and social interaction.

Teacher objective
Getting the campers to enjoy yoga as an activity, to work together cooperatively, and to alleviate some of the crabbiness of the campers because it is raining—again. After each activity, take a minute to reflect on the activity, letting all students contribute.

Yoga space

Carpeted area. Not a great deal of room, but big enough for the students to work cooperatively in partners and groups.

Equipment needed for this lesson

Relaxation script, music and CD player, and blindfolds.

Introductory or opening exercise

Colored breath. (5 minutes)

Warm-up

1. Trusting circle.

   ▨ Student reflection: How can we work together to build trust?

2. Trust walk.

   ▨ Student reflection: How can we help each other during this exercise? (15 minutes)

Workout

Students work in partners doing poses.

   ▨ Partner bridge.

   ▸ Student reflection: How can this activity be made easier?

   ▨ Upward-facing boats.

   ▸ Student reflection: How can we work to support each other in this activity?

   ▨ Lizard snoozing on a rock.

   ▸ Student reflection: How can we communicate safety while doing this activity?

   ▨ Back-to-back partner poses: Standing back to back, partners do triangle, warrior II, and tree with their backs each supporting the other, or they can each move in the opposite direction and still support each other.

   ▨ Partners create a made-up pose and give it a fun name.

   ▨ Show the group a pose you came up with. (15 minutes)

Floor exercises and cool-down

Tell students to do hammock pose while pretending they are at their favorite spot at the camp.

Relaxation

Relaxation script with relaxing music. (12 minutes)

Closing

Ask the students, "How can you work together as a team for our upcoming challenge?" For example, climbing a wall, putting up a tent, going on a scavenger hunt, or doing another camp competition. (3 minutes)

Brief reflection

How did yoga work as a camp activity? How was the group process enhanced through the partner and group activities? Are there elements of yoga that can be brought up when the group does other camp activities that require cooperation, patience, and listening?

Sample Lesson Plan for Grades 9-12 or Athletes

This lesson plan is for older students in high school or on an athletic team. It includes "mix-ins," or poses that can be inserted into sun salutations. These poses are held for one to five breaths, and then the sun salutation continues. For example, a warrior pose with the right foot in front could be mixed in, or inserted into, the traditional sun salutation and held for five breaths. The sun salutation flowing poses would continue with the warrior pose mixed in again, this time with the left leg forward. This allows for physically active yoga classes through integration of the cardiorespiratory activity of the sun salutation with the strength and flexibility poses of the mix-ins.

Date of lesson, group, amount of time, setting
Group of 12 students at a 50-minute drop-in yoga class at the teen center.

Purpose or theme of the lesson
Taking a yoga class as a voluntary activity at a local teen center.

Physical education standard addressed
Standard 6: Values physical activity for health, enjoyment, challenge, self-expression, and social interaction.

Teacher objective
To teach a yoga class that helps teens build a repertoire of sun salutations and poses for their continued participation in yoga.

Yoga space
Activity space at a teen center.

Equipment needed for this lesson
CD of yoga music that is popular for teens (see resource section); yoga mats for each student.

Introductory or opening exercise
1. Breath exercise with posture alignment: Calming breath five counts in and five counts out.
2. Alternative nostril breathing. Ask students to set an intention for their yoga practice. "What do you want from your practice today?" (3 minutes)

Warm-up
1. Cross-legged seated pose flow sequence: Inhale and reach both arms up. Exhale and twist the belly button, chest, and arms to the right. Inhale and sweep both arms back up to the sky, and on the next exhale, twist to the left. Inhale and sweep both arms back up to the sky. Exhale and reach both arms into a side bend to the right—right hand can reach to the floor. Inhale back up and on the next exhale, reach into a side bend to the left. On the inhale, reach both arms to the sky and reach forward into a cross-legged forward fold and hold. Do five balloon breaths while holding the cross-legged forward fold. (3 minutes)
2. Repeat the whole sequence, switching legs so the opposite leg is now folded in front in the cross-legged seated pose. (3 minutes)

Workout, part 1: Core strength table flow sequence

1. On the floor, start in table. Inhale: cow pose. Exhale: downward-facing dog. Inhale: plank. Exhale: downward-facing dog. Inhale: cow pose.

2. Finish: child pose. (3 minutes)

Workout, part 2: Balancing table flow sequence

1. Start in table. The right arm reaches forward and the left leg reaches back; both are held at hip height or lower—hold eye gaze on a focus point (dhristi), keeping the breath strong and full.

2. Lower and step left foot back into a runner's lunge, balancing on the right knee. Bring the torso and the arms up, and come into kneeling warrior. Hold for five breaths. Release into child pose. Come into balancing table on the other side, and this time come into a runner's lunge with the right leg back, balancing on the left bent knee into kneeling. Do warrior, both arms to the sky.

3. Finish: child pose. (5 minutes)

Workout, part 3: Sun salutations

1. Start in mountain. Salute the sun, reaching both arms strongly to the ceiling. Forward dive into standing forward fold. Step the left foot back into a runner's lunge, then add the right foot and hold the body in plank. Slowly lower the whole body down to the floor, and come into cobra. Push the body up and back into downward-facing dog. Step the right foot forward between the hands while keeping the left foot back in a runner's lunge. Step the left foot forward, and hold in standing forward fold. Reverse forward dive. Salute the sun. Finish: mountain.

2. Repeat sequence on other side. (12 minutes)

Mix-Ins

During the sun salutations, poses can be mixed in and held for a specific number of breaths. From step back into lunge, do the mix-in pose, which can be held for five breaths, and then step back to lunge and follow the sequence of plank, lower to cobra, downward-facing dog, and lunge, and then do the mix-in on the other side. Finish the rest of the sun salutation.

Mix-In Strength Poses

- Warriors: I, II, III, reverse
- Extended side angle
- Chair

Mix-In Balance Poses

- Tree
- Standing bow
- Eagle
- Lighthouse

Any pose can be mixed in. Have fun mixing it up!

Workout, part 4: Standing poses

Standing wide-angle forward fold pose, tree pose, eagle pose. (3 minutes)

Floor exercises and cool-down

Seated forward fold using a strap or towel. Boat. Butterfly. Superhero. Bridge. (8 minutes)

Relaxation

1. Lying spinal twist.

2. Relaxation pose. Use relaxing music and a script for relaxation (7 minutes; see chapter 6).

Closing

Cross-legged seated pose. Say to the students, "Come back to the breath exercises we practiced at the beginning. Check in with the intention you set for your practice today. Take a moment to reflect on the positive changes in your body and mind from your yoga practice. Does anyone want to share?" (3 minutes)

Brief reflection

How can this class be even more special and the yoga space set up so that this activity is important and respected by teens as an important activity to balance their lives? How can you encourage participation and have the students be active learners? Is there music or poetry the students can bring, art they want to use to decorate the space, journals they can bring? Can there be theme days or ways to encourage the teens to bring a friend?

INDOOR RECESS YOGA

Recess allows for peer interaction, a break from academics, meaningful play, and a way to burn off energy. Many schools that canceled recess for the sake of more academic time have reinstated it because students need this valuable time. When the weather or other circumstances require recess to be indoors, many teachers are at a loss for a good activity to do. Unfortunately, indoor recess often becomes free time where students passively sit or zone out on electronics, computers, or video games. Yoga can be a great activity to practice in the classroom. What is described here does not need to be reserved for recess but can also be used as a mini yoga break for about 10 minutes in duration.

Where can you find yoga time?

- Between classes or subjects as a transition and break
- A transition between recess and coming back into the learning space
- A transition from the lunch room back to the classroom
- In a counseling session, allowing the student to find time to feel grounded and centered
- Group facilitation to allow the group to work cooperatively
- On a special day: Friday mornings or afternoons; a field day activity

The following are examples of yoga games that can be played while students are at their desks or standing on a mat when moving around the room is not feasible (e.g., a classroom without a lot of space).

ACTION STORY

▪ Indoor Recess

Make up a story that has a lot of action words and poses infused into it. The students have to listen carefully, and when there is an action or pose word, they do the action or pose.

Here is an example of a story: "Today we are going on an adventure. Put on your hiking boots [action] and your hat [action] and backpack [action]. Are you ready? We are going to the jungle! We are slowly hiking [action] up the mountain to get to our jungle. We have to hop over big rocks [action], and what's that? We see birds overhead [look up]. It's a flamingo [do standing bow pose]. OK, let's keep going, but we need to drink some water [action]. It is getting a little chilly, and you are shivering [action]. Open up your backpack and put on your jacket [action]." And so on . . . (5 minutes)

"AS IF" GAME

▪ Indoor Recess

To get students to burn off some energy at their desks, play the "as if" game.

- Jog *as if* you were running on the moon.
- Move your arms *as if* you were a train going up a long hill (slow) and then coming down the hill (fast!).
- Walk *as if* your legs and arms were made of chocolate pudding.
- Jump in place *as if* you were a popcorn kernel.
- Reach to the sky *as if* you were grabbing balloons.
- Paint a beautiful picture *as if* your head were a paint brush.
- Swim *as if* you were in a bowl of yellow Jell-O.
- Move your feet *as if* you were on an ice skating rink with no skates.

Mix things up in the "as if" game by adding in yoga poses:

- Stand *as if* you were a big, strong tree more than 100 years old (tree pose).
- Stand *as if* you were in a flock of seagulls on the beach (standing bow pose). (5 minutes)

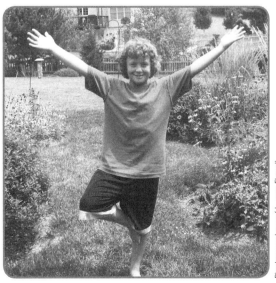

Photo courtesy of Lucas Flavell.

Student standing as if he is a strong, old tree.

MORNING ROUTINE

▪ **Indoor Recess**

Each student makes up her own sequence of favorite poses. There can be a limit to the number of poses included so it does not get too long, complicated, or tedious. The sequence can be done silently or with a singsong, rhyme, or music. Students each get a turn to lead her sequence and call it a special name (e.g., Sara's Silly Wake-up).

YOGA UNIT PLAN

The yoga unit plan is a sequential plan for starting with basic yoga poses. With each subsequent lesson, more poses are introduced or more-challenging poses are included. In a community setting (e.g., a YMCA), students might sign up for a 4-, 6-, or 8-week course where a unit plan could be used. However, what often happens is not everyone is there for every single class, so poses may need to be reviewed again and again. A word of advice: Although you want to keep students motivated and engaged, yoga has been around for thousands of years, using the same basic poses practiced over and over again. This is what yoga is—a practice— and students must be encouraged to understand that yoga is not something we master or are entertained by but rather something we can practice and learn from each time we do it.

Another way a unit plan can be utilized is as part of a physical education curriculum where a week is devoted to yoga. Table 5.2 is a simple example for middle school through teens of a progression that could be done over a series of days or classes, such as week-to-week classes. The idea is to keep building on poses they are familiar with and then adding a few more challenges each class. Provide students with as much practice as possible, and mix it up so the challenges are fresh and fun.

YOGA LESSON AND UNIT PLANS FOR SPECIAL GROUPS

This section provides information, strategies, and best practices of how to introduce and implement yoga in various settings and groups.

Yoga Workout for Student-Athletes

Yoga is a great activity for athletes, and your athletes will be surprised at just how many of their favorite athletes and sports teams use yoga as a training tool. Yoga is a valuable activity for athletes that helps with stretching, flexibility, balance, and coordination, which are all important elements of physical training, but it is even more valuable as a mental training tool. Students can learn to use their breath to calm down and focus in competition; keep their focus during distractions, such as yelling fans or hearing troublesome comments from opponents; or conserve their energy in endurance events so they remain fresh and alert.

This sample workout offers recommended strength and balance poses along with mental exercises that have proven especially beneficial when working with student-athletes.

TABLE 5.2 Sample of a One-Week Unit Plan

	Day 1	Day 2	Day 3	Day 4	Day 5
Warm-up	Mountain Standing quarter moon	Review from day 1 New: Standing back bend	Review from days 1 and 2 New: Standing forward fold	Review from days 1-3 New: Standing wide-angle forward fold	Review from days 1-4 and put into different sequence patterns New: Standing chest stretcher
Workout	Chair pose Warrior 1 Warrior 2 Triangle	Review from day 1 New: Reverse warrior Warrior 3	Review from days 1 and 2 New: Tree Downward-facing dog	Review from days 1-3 New: Extended side angle Eagle	Review from days 1-4 and put into different sequence patterns New: Standing bow Lighthouse
Floor exercises and cool-down	Seated forward fold Butterfly Happy baby pose	Review from day 1 New: Cobra	Review from days 1 and 2 New: Boat Bridge Superhero	Review from days 1-3 New: Camel Bow	Review from days 1-4 New: Balancing table
Relaxation	Relaxation pose	Happy baby	Nose to knees	Lying spinal twist stretch	Kermit the Frog, fetal

Warm-up
- Balloon breath with affirmations. Example: "I am getting stronger every day."
- Guided imagination. Example: imagining the perfect play or execution of a skill.
- Meditation. Example: the strengths the student brings to the team.

Workout
Flowing sun salutations with mix-ins: warriors, tree, eagle, standing bow, kneeling warrior, triangle, standing wide-angle forward fold

Core strength poses
Boat, bridge, plank, side plank, cobra, superhero, upward-facing dog, three-legged dog, downward-facing dog, slow-motion abdominal curls

Floor exercises and cool-down
Seated forward fold, table pose, turtle pose, rock the baby, lying spinal twist

Relaxation
- Relaxation scripts including inspiring quotes
- Self-affirmation meditation, where students write an affirming statement on a note card
- Gratitude meditation (see chapter 8)

Yoga for At-Risk Youth: Juvenile Justice and Homeless Students

Yoga has been found to be useful in treating and working with at-risk youth. Street Yoga, based in Portland, Oregon, provides a program called Safe Space, which includes yoga, meals, and medical care for homeless and other at-risk youth. Another example is the Sisterhood Project, a 6-week stress-management and mentoring program that paired at-risk high school girls with female university student mentors as they engaged in weekly stress-management activities together. This group of partners enjoyed activities such as journal writing, healthy snacks, relaxing music, massage, spa treatments, and yoga. There is so much we can offer at-risk students at little or no cost. Spend some time looking at the recommended Web sites in the resource section to find more inspiring ideas on ways to reach all of your students.

Following is an example of a 40-minute yoga class and yoga art done with 12 at-risk teenage girls in a residential program.

Introductory or opening exercise

1. Cross-legged seated pose: The theme for the class is communication. Discuss and review guidelines in yoga that support good communication in everyday situations.

2. Breath exercise: alternate nostril breathing.

3. Setting of intention for today's practice. (5 minutes)

Warm-up

Cross-legged seated pose flow sequence (3 minutes)

Workout

Standing goddess sequence: All poses in the sequence are held for five breaths—this can be repeated several times depending on the time available.

Standing frog pose with arms in cactus. Open out to the right in warrior II, then triangle to the right, runner's lunge to the right; come into standing wide-angle forward fold and hold. Move to the left into runner's lunge, come up into triangle to the left, then warrior II to the left, and finish in standing frog. Repeat the whole sequence now, starting with warrior II to the left and so on. (5 minutes)

Floor exercises and cool-down

Boat, cobra, bridge (5 minutes)

Relaxation

Relaxation pose and gratitude meditation (7 minutes)

Yoga Art Activity

Form an inclusive circle, doing alternate nostril breathing and then checking in with intention.

Students in pairs trace around their partners to make a large outline of their favorite yoga pose and then color it in. These will be used to decorate the yoga space. (10 minutes)

Closing

Students share their yoga art with the group. (5 minutes)

Yoga and Students With Depression

Students with depression may need a yoga class with poses that are more restorative and soothing in nature. The poses included here are very soothing to the nervous system, and along with deep, relaxed breathing, they help students improve mood states and feel calmer and more in control. The following is a recommended sequence of poses for this yoga class.

Warm-up
Reclining butterfly, knees to nose pose (single leg to chest, switch, and then hold onto both knees), happy baby pose

Workout
Downward-facing dog, standing forward fold, standing bow

Floor exercises and cool-down
Seated twist, bridge

Relaxation
Legs up against the wall, relaxation pose, Kermit the Frog pose

Yoga and Students With Attention-Deficit/Hyperactivity Disorder

Yoga is an effective tool when working with students with attention problems. The type of poses used with this population is not as important as the instructional methods. Yoga helps these students calm down and feel self-control. The instructional methods need to reinforce the following attributes that students can develop:

- Feeling centered and grounded by having established rules to follow
- Focusing on breathing and checking in with their bodies
- Instead of feeding off of and competing with the mood and energy of others, encouraging students with ADHD to do what is best for them (e.g., taking breaks and learning to relax)

Some interesting research has been done on students with attention disorders stabilized with medications. Yoga was found to be an effective treatment for stabilizing emotions and reducing oppositional behavior of young males (10.63 mean years of age). Participants took 20 weekly sessions partnered with daily home practice (Jensen & Kenny, 2004).

The sample lesson plan for this group includes traditional activities balanced with a meditation activity and a relaxation activity.

Introductory or opening exercise
Hot air balloon breath

Warm-up
Sun salutations

Workout
Yoga games: oodles of noodles and yoga jive five yoga station

Floor exercises and cool-down
Another five-activity station that includes floor exercises (e.g., rowing boat, bridge, Jessica's soup pose, superhero, and reverse plank)

Relaxation
Relaxation pose

Closing
Counting breaths meditation and peace train

Yoga and Students in Wheelchairs

Yoga can be easily adapted for students in wheelchairs or who need to use a chair during a yoga class. Students can also work with partners and participate in the creative problem-solving activities. Instead of seeing an accessibility issue as a problem, see it as a chance to work together to make the class fun, engaging, inclusive, challenging, and meaningful for all students! As you plan your yoga lesson, have a chair handy to practice the instruction and possible modifications before teaching the class so that without skipping a beat, you have modifications ready to go.

SUMMARY

Good teaching involves good planning, but also remember that the art of teaching and the art of teaching yoga are about being flexible and open to whatever might present itself as a teachable moment.

The next chapter provides instruction on helping students learn to breathe correctly and gives ideas for students to learn to relax—both lifelong skills.

chapter 6

Breathing and Relaxation Exercises

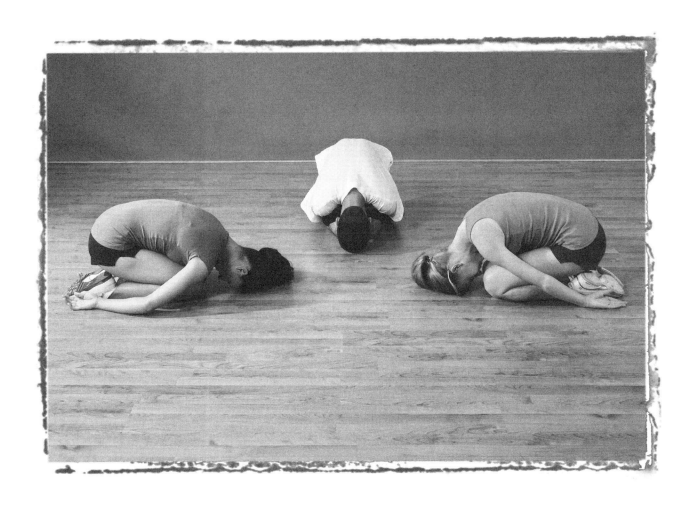

*T*his chapter provides ideas for teaching the most important skills of yoga for healthy and balanced living. These skills include helping students shift their attention and energy appropriately to yoga or any activity and helping students develop their self-efficacy (i.e., their belief in their own ability to do tasks) and practice proactive methods to calm and relax themselves.

TRANSITIONS INTO YOGA PRACTICE

Transitions refer to exercises typically done with students at both the beginning and the end of class. As students come from other classes or activities, they may be in a hurry or their attention may still be on what they were doing before. Students need to make the transition from the busy outside world to a place to settle down and enjoy yoga practice.

How the class ends is equally important. The ending of the class should allow the students to assimilate all they have learned in their yoga class and prepare them to transition into whatever presents itself in the rest of their day in a calm and relaxed attitude. In beginning a yoga class, breath and transition exercises are used to help the students make the transition from what they were doing before yoga to the yoga session. The section on the gift of relaxation provides relaxation exercises that allow the students to assimilate all they have learned in yoga that day and to approach the next activity in their day refreshed, calm, and centered. The relaxation section also includes the use of guided imagery and meditation as tools for relaxation. Throughout this chapter are infusion ideas, which are ways to enrich the learning experience by infusing other topics and subjects into the yoga activities.

BEGINNING THE YOGA CLASS: BREATHING EXERCISES

The beginning of yoga class is a critical step to a wonderful learning experience for students. The opening may need to be longer if the students have just come from a hectic class or are just plain crabby. Including relaxing music or a soundtrack of ocean wave sounds, birds chirping, or other nature sounds can bring a soothing aspect into opening the yoga class.

One of the easiest ways to start class is with a breath exercise. In yoga, both the inhalation and exhalation are through the nose, with the lips together. Breathing through the nose allows for better control; better focus; and fuller, relaxed breaths while humidifying and filtering the air. If a student has a cold or allergies, please modify these guidelines—breathing through the mouth is fine. Learning to breathe correctly should never be forced or uncomfortable but a process toward gradually making the breath slower, deeper, and easier.

Breath Exercises for All Students

Teaching breath exercises at the beginning of class sets the stage for authentic yoga. Breath exercises are the general opening exercises to use with all student groups. The most important gift of yoga is its foundation: breath. Breath is the bridge between the body and mind. Becoming mindful of the breath and learning how to make the breath more focused, full, and relaxed at the start of each class will help the students have a motivating and wonderful yoga experience and can be one of the valuable lifestyle skills students can learn, as it will influence everything they do both in class and outside of class.

BALLOON BREATH

(can also be called three-part breath, yoga breath, or Dirga breath)

▪ **Breath**

This breath exercise helps students realize that their breath moves in their bodies in three directions:

- Direction 1 moves the breath into the front and back of the body and starts in the belly; the breath is felt in the belly area (front) and lower torso (back).
- Direction 2 moves the breath out into the ribs using the intercostal muscles; the breath expands the chest cavity from side to side.
- Direction 3 moves the breath up into the heart space, drawing the breath from the bottom of the spine all the way up to the top of the clavicles.

Start

Begin in a cross-legged seated pose.

1. Start with some deep, relaxing breaths, and feel the breath as it enters the belly. Remind students to feel the breath fill up the belly and lower back. Place the hands on the belly to feel the breath fill it up.

2. Bring the hands up and place them on the ribs, feeling the breath expand the ribs as if they are fanning out to the side.

3. Place the fingertips just under the collarbones. Remind students to feel the breath start deep in the belly, and feel it as it moves from the bottom of the belly all the way up to the collarbones.

4. Allow time for students to notice the breath as it fills up the belly, expands out to the ribs, and draws all the way up to the chest. Say to them, "Inhale: belly, ribs, chest. Exhale: chest, ribs, belly."

5. Tell students to pretend they are blowing up a big balloon in the body and to make it as big as they can. Cue them by saying, "Ready; start blowing up the balloon in the belly, the ribs, all the way up to the top of the chest. OK, now slowly let the air out of the balloon by slowly exhaling the breath out of the chest, ribs, and now finally the belly. Did you get all the air out? Bring the belly button to your spine to get all the air out."

Variation A

Balloon breath can be practiced in child pose, against a wall, with a partner's hands on the lower back, back to back against a partner, and with a Beanie Baby on the lower abdomen.

Variation B: Hot Air Balloon Breath
(can also be called pump it up breath)

Hot air balloon breath is a great way to help students get energized for yoga class. This exercise helps students connect to the inhalation phase of breathing through stretching upward to energize the body and conversely connect to the exhalation phase of the breath with a forward fold to help relax the body.
Start from a standing position.

1. Ask the students to crouch down low and, on the inhale, start filling up their hot air balloons by slowly standing up until they are standing with rounded arms reaching overhead. Hold the hot air balloon up in the sky for three breaths.
2. With the exhale, the balloon deflates. Tell students to release the breath and body by slowly crouching down like a rag doll. "Just hang there with no muscles or bones to hold you up; just stay loose and relaxed."
3. Repeat.

Variation C: Wave Breath

Start by lying prone with the legs straight out, arms along the sides of the body.

1. Place a small Beanie Baby, a small stuffed toy, or an eye bag just below the belly button.
2. Seal the mouth and breathe through the nose.
3. With the inhale, breathe into the belly, and watch the Beanie Baby rise.
4. With the exhale, let the belly relax, and watch the Beanie Baby gently sink.
5. Tell students, "Try this a few more times, and watch the Beanie Baby 'swim' up and down on the wave of the breath."

Variation D (for older students)

Ask the class to imagine the breath as a wave gently coming into shore. Imagine the wave building and coming into the beach with the inhale and slowly coming away, or receding, from the shore with the exhale.

Variation E

Another way to help students use their breathing muscles is through feather blowing. Blow a feather or Nerf ball (soft ball) into the center of the circle to develop belly breathing. Be careful students do not overexert themselves by making this into a competition; it is a focus and concentration exercise.

BELLY BREATH

▪ **Breath**

In this breathing exercise, students become familiar with the diaphragm muscle and how to breathe correctly, both for yoga practice and to relax. In belly breath (see figure 6.1), the hands are placed on the lower abdomen and will lift upon the inhalation as the belly fills with air; the diaphragm pulls downward, allowing the lungs to fill with more air deep into the lower parts of the lungs. During the exhalation, the diaphragm relaxes and the hands will gently fall as the belly gently drops.

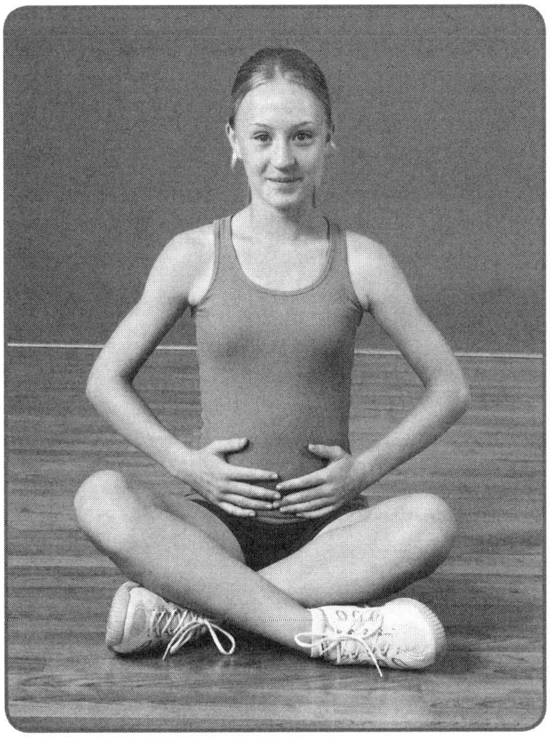

FIGURE 6.1 Belly breath.

Start

Begin in a cross-legged seated pose.

1. Keeping the back strong, lift the heart space, shoulder blades back and down. The ears should be aligned over the shoulders, with the chin parallel to the ground.

2. Remind students to keep the belly area as relaxed and soft as possible. Place the palms of the hands on the lower belly, below the belly button.

3. Start to notice the movement of the breath. The hands will gently move up upon the inhale and slowly drop upon the exhale.

Variation

Lie on the back with the knees bent and feet flat on the floor or legs extended.

Infusion Idea

Discuss the importance of oxygen to living things, clean air, and using the belly breath when we need to get calm and centered.

BUNNY NOSE

(can also be called whale spout breath or dragon breath)

▪ **Breath**

This exercise helps students learn to breathe through the nose, which is much more relaxing and controlled than mouth breathing (see figure 6.2).

Start

Begin in a cross-legged seated pose.

1. Take a big breath through the nose, with the mouth closed.
2. Slowly breathe out through the nose in three to five short bursts, telling the students to "wrinkle up the nose like a bunny."

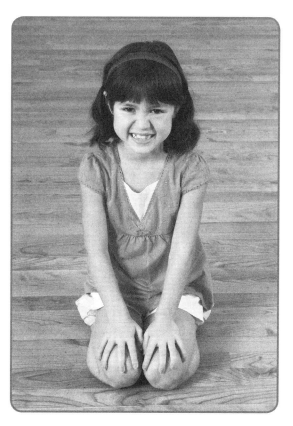

FIGURE 6.2   Bunny nose.

Variation

Use the image of a whale spout releasing breath or a dragon breathing out fire from its nose.

GREEN MEANIES

▪ **Breath**

This exercise brings in colors to add a creative element.

Start

Begin by lying on the back with the legs extended.

1. Cue students by saying, "Imagine green meanies in your belly—these meanies are all the problems you might be having right now, and you need to get rid of them. Now imagine holes in the bottom of your feet, and with your breath you are going to let those meanies ooze out. Imagine that every time you exhale, the green meanies are pushed out through the holes in the bottom of your feet."
2. Tell students to exhale a few more times to make sure the last of the "green meanies" are gone.

HEART BREATH

■ **Breath**

This breath exercise helps students connect with the wonderful qualities their hearts represent: being loving, being a good friend, listening, caring, having gratitude, and sharing feelings.

Start

This exercise can be done anywhere: sitting, standing, or waiting in line.

1. Take a few moments to connect with the breath, and make it relaxed and peaceful.

2. Bring your attention to the heart space, and imagine breathing in and out of the heart space.

3. Ask students to remember a time when they felt happy and full of joy.

4. Say to the class, "Imagine you are there again right now, and feel what it was like to feel this good. Enjoy this special place in your heart for a few more breaths."

6. Remind students that whenever they need a break, they can take a heart breath. All they need to do is take a few moments, breathe relaxed and slow breaths in and out of the heart space, and remember that special place in their hearts.

Infusion Idea

Students can share their special heartfelt memories with the class or through journals or artwork.

HUMMINGBIRD BREATH

(can also be called buzzing bee breath)

■ **Breath**

The soothing of a humming sound can help relax the body.

Start

Make a soft humming or buzzing sound in the lower part of the back of the throat during exhalation through the nose, with the mouth sealed. You can try making the sound have different octaves. It is important to keep this breath down in the lower part of the throat and not up in the mouth, which can become uncomfortable. Try for 30 to 60 seconds, but the noise you make should be steady and calm like a hummingbird in nature.

LION'S ROAR

■ **Breath**

Sometimes your students need to let out frustration, let out trapped energy, or hear their voices. If the students come into yoga class with a lot of pent-up energy, lion's roar can help burn some of it off (see figure 6.3).

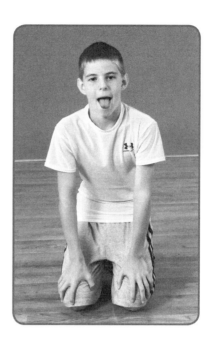

FIGURE 6.3 Lion's roar.

Start

Kneel on the floor, sitting back on the heels. Hands rest on the thighs.

1. Inhale through the nose.
2. Exhale and overexaggerate a lion's roar by stretching and sticking out the tongue, making all of the face stretch (even the ears!), and while opening up the mouth wide, make a big, long, and fierce roar sound deep from the belly like a lion.
3. Try it two more times, making the roar come from deep down in the belly muscles so it is a ROAR instead of from the lungs and throat, which comes out like a scream.
4. Take a big yawn with such a big stretch for the face that even the ears stretch back, like the ears of a big cat.

Infusion Idea

Students make up poses that look like their favorite animals, then parade around the room in a circle.

PEACE TRAIN

■ **Breath**

This exercise emphasizes the importance of knowing that peace begins with each of us.

Start

Begin by sitting tall and strong in a cross-legged seated pose.

1. Breathe through the nose, and imagine a shiny bright white light at the heart center. Continue to breathe in smoothly and steadily through the nose, and imagine this light shining strongly and brightly to all of the body—the face, the torso, the back, the legs, the arms, the hands, and the head.
2. Say to the class, "Now let this bright white light shine and fill up this room, this school, this neighborhood, this state, this country, the world! This light represents peace, and peace begins with each of us."

Infusion Idea

Discuss how we can be more peaceful and live more peacefully.

QUIETING BREATH

(can also be called chilling breath)

▪ **Breath**

This exercise brings in colors to add a creative element to address the whole child.

Start

Begin by lying down or assuming a seated position.

1. Inhale with the arms reaching overhead, and tell students to pretend they are inhaling cool blue air.
2. Slowly lower the arms back down, pretending to exhale warm red air.
3. Repeat.

RELEASE AND RECHARGE BREATH

(can also be called R & R breath)

▪ **Breath**

This exercise focuses on exhalation, which is the most relaxing part of the breath.

Start

Begin by lying down or assuming a seated position.

1. Inhale and slowly exhale and release tension from the face, neck, shoulders, core, and legs.
2. Inhale and slowly exhale and release any worries, crankiness, fatigue, or negative thoughts or feelings.
3. Inhale and slowly exhale and picture the whole body and mind feeling recharged and full of positive energy.
4. Take as many breaths as needed to completely release and relax the body and mind and to feel the body recharge.

Infusion Idea

Ask students what makes them feel recharged and what makes them feel relaxed. Students can share their own special positive ways to recharge, such as eating a healthy snack or quietly reading a book.

Breathing Exercises for Older Students

The breath exercises already introduced can be used with all students, with wording modifications to meet the students' developmental stages. Using age-appropriate vocabulary allows the students to understand the feeling of what you want them to experience. An example is using the word *belly* with younger children; with older students, explaining the mechanics behind why you want them to adopt diaphragmatic breathing will be more meaningful and appropriate. The following breath exercises are more advanced for older students and can also be used with student-athletes.

ALTERNATE NOSTRIL BREATHING

■ **Breathing exercise for older students**

Alternate nostril breathing can help clear the mind and facilitate using the right and left hemispheres of the brain (see figure 6.4).

Start

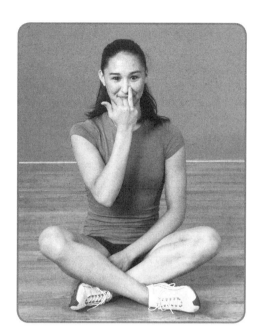

FIGURE 6.4 Alternate nostril breathing.

1. The thumb and index finger of the right hand are used alternately to close off a nostril while the air is inhaled or exhaled through the other nostril.

2. Slowly inhale through the right nostril as you pinch off, or close, the left nostril with the index finger. Hold both nostrils for one count.

3. Slowly release the left nostril, and exhale through the left nostril as you pinch off the right nostril with the thumb.

4. Inhale through the left nostril (the right nostril is still pinched off), hold both nostrils for one count, and now release the thumb from the right nostril. Exhale slowly through the right nostril as you close off the left nostril with the thumb.

5. It will take a few cycles to get into the rhythm of this breath exercise, but students will find they are more awake and energized as they get used to it.

UJJAYI BREATH

(can also be called Darth Vader or ocean-sounding breath)

■ **Breathing exercise for older students**

This breath is commonly used in yoga to help remain focused, especially during challenging poses. The sound is very soothing to the nervous system, and with the toning of the throat muscles, the breath can be controlled to prevent hyperventilating when stressed.

1. Begin the exercise by saying, "To first understand the sound you are trying to create, bring your palm up to your mouth and exhale on it as if you are trying to fog up a mirror. Try this again on the inhale. You will notice that this really dries out the throat. We will now make this noise, but with the lips sealed."

2. Inhale and exhale through the nose, and constrict the throat muscles as if whispering or fogging a mirror—the sound can start out as a soft snore but can be amplified.

3. Students may try the sound only on the inhale or exhale and master that and then try to do it on both the inhale and exhale.

THE GIFT OF RELAXATION

Beautiful endings happen when the end of class includes an extended relaxation period of 5 to 10 minutes, where you integrate all that was done in class to assimilate the benefits. Real relaxation is achieved through focus and concentration, although this may seem counterintuitive. The students practice mindfulness by focusing on specific sensations in the body, the feeling in the muscles, and the ebb and flow of the breath. Remember, relaxation exercises can be used throughout the class to rejuvenate and to balance the more vigorous or active poses. Students can use relaxation poses and exercises to reenergize after school for homework or other activities; before bed to help them sleep better; whenever they are sick or feeling run down to help improve immune function; and whenever they feel anxious, angry, or stressed.

Relaxation Exercises

At the end of class, depending on the age group and time allowed, there should be some kind of culminating experience that allows the body and mind to absorb the yoga practice. Therefore, providing time for relaxation is critical for all students. Terms such as *quiet time, relaxation time*, or *Sleeping Beauty pose* may be substituted and may be a more-appropriate interpretation for our students. Other ideas to facilitate relaxation include reading a short poem or playing a musical selection. Any ritual or tradition can be used as a wonderful way to end yoga practice. It is important to tune into students' body language and energy. Often students will move in intuitive ways that can be picked up on as the exact right thing to do in that moment for relaxation.

Younger children can bring a favorite stuffed animal to hug to help them settle into relaxation. Instructors can place an eye bag over the students' eyes or gently massage their feet. Keeping a supply of blankets and laying the blankets over the students can help them relax, as well as turning down the lights if possible. As discussed in chapter 3, modulating the voice for relaxation time can help cue children that it is time to settle down.

The whole class may have a hard time settling down and making adjustments, so suggesting alternative relaxation poses can help. For example, students may find lying on their backs too difficult and can be encouraged to lie on their tummies in Kermit the Frog pose (one knee bent and the other straight) or in fetal pose (lying on the side with knees curled up). It is important to encourage students to seek out these poses when they become tired or overwhelmed. As discussed in chapter 3, students should not come out of or stop a pose and sit and watch other students. Students need to find what is called a restorative pose to help them relax, get their energy back, or just calm down. It is recommended that students close their eyes during relaxation exercises, but some students do not feel comfortable doing this in class, so suggest it but do not push it.

BEACH BALLS

▪ **Relaxation**

This pose is a great self-massage and relaxation for the lower back.

Start

Begin by lying on the back.

1. Bring the knees to the chest (nose to knees pose), and hold onto the tops of the knees or underneath the knees at the hamstrings.
2. Gently rock side to side and front to back without letting go of the knees.

CHAIR RELAXATION

▪ **Relaxation**

There may be times when students cannot lie down on the floor for relaxation, so helping them learn to relax in a chair is valuable.

Start

Begin while seated in a chair.

1. Tell the students to be still and very quiet as they settle into their chairs and find a position that allows them to rest.
2. Listen to the breath, and soften and relax the head and neck, the shoulders and arms, the heart, the belly, the back, the legs, and the feet.

CHILD POSE

▪ **Relaxation**

This is a very relaxing pose that students can use at any time during yoga to rest and be quiet. If at any time during a class a student feels overwhelmed or tired, child pose is a wonderful pose to find respite and relaxation (see figure 6.5).

Start

Begin on hands and knees or kneeling on the floor.

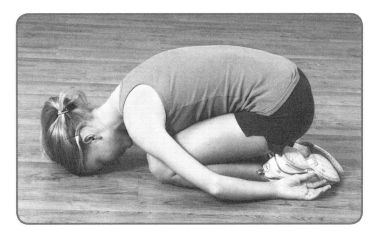

FIGURE 6.5 Child pose.

1. Sit back so the gluteals rest on the heels, with toes either curled under or flat.

2. Fold forward, and bring the arms around alongside the body, resting the forehead on the floor in front or on the platform of one fist stacked on top of the other.

HAMMOCK

▪ **Relaxation**

This pose allows for the lower back to relax and feel supported by the floor (see figure 6.6).

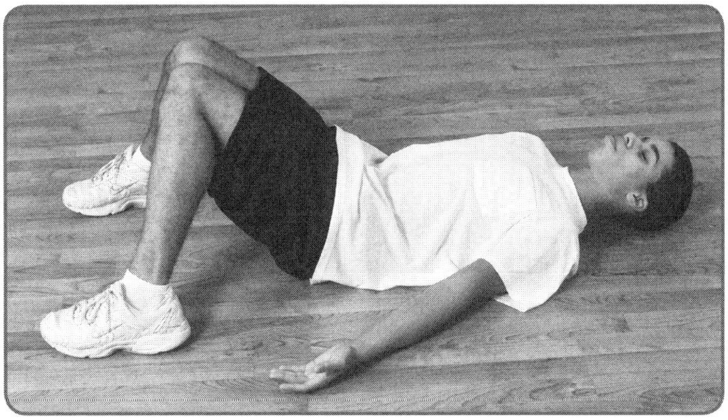

Start

Begin by lying on the back, with the feet about 1 foot (30 centimeters) apart while keeping the knees together, allowing the lower back to settle into the floor.

Infusion Idea

FIGURE 6.6 Hammock pose.

Ask the students to visualize slowly lowering themselves into a hammock. At first when using a hammock, we may not let all our weight be supported by the hammock, but as we relax, the body slowly relaxes so we can rest effortlessly.

KERMIT THE FROG

▦ **Relaxation**

The pose is very intuitive for relaxing when we are on our abdomens. Drawing one knee up is a comfortable and relaxing pose (see figure 6.7).

Start

Begin prone on the belly.

1. Draw one knee up in line with the hips, making the shape of a frog leg.
2. The other leg remains straight, and the upper body can rest on a pillow or folded blanket, with the head turned to the side.

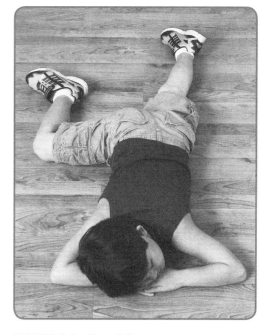

FIGURE 6.7 Kermit the Frog pose.

LEGS UP AGAINST THE WALL

▦ **Relaxation**

This is a great exercise to help students quiet down; it gives their circulation a rest as well.

Start

Sit down close against a wall, and slowly lower the back to the floor as you gently swing the legs up to rest against the wall. Let the legs fall slightly apart and rest (see figure 6.8).

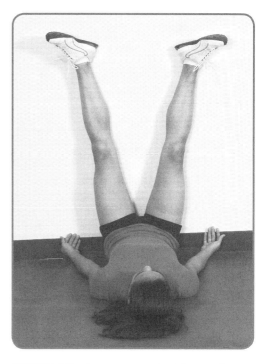

FIGURE 6.8 Legs up against the wall.

LYING GENTLE SPINE-TWIST POSE

(can also be called angels in the snow)

■ **Relaxation**

This pose allows for a wonderful gentle stretch and twisting of the spine in order to let the whole spine feel open and relaxed (see figure 6.9).

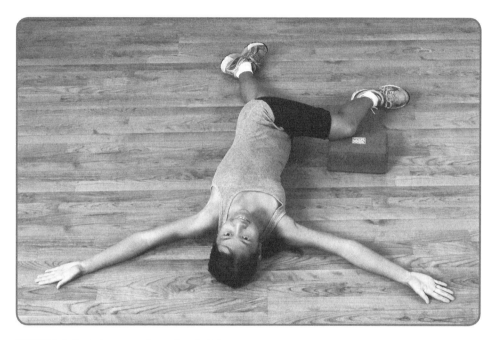

FIGURE 6.9   Lying gentle spine-twist pose.

Start

Begin by lying on the back.

1. Bring the right knee in to the chest, with the left leg extended along the floor. Arms come out straight to the sides in what is referred to as airplane arms.

2. With the left hand, slowly bring the right knee over to the left side of the body to rest on the floor or on a blanket or yoga block. Allow as much as possible for both shoulders to settle and relax into the floor, and keep the right arm reaching out to the side with the palm up. It is not necessary for the left shoulder to touch the floor, but let it relax as much as possible.

Variation

Both knees can be bent. Tell students that if the pose is not comfortable, they can go into fetal pose.

MACARONI TEST

▪ **Relaxation**

Set up the exercise by saying, "When you open a box of macaroni and cheese, the noodles are hard. But once you cook them, they are soft, floppy, and warm. We are going to make our bodies like warm, gooey macaroni and cheese. We'll test your body to make sure it is cooked just right."

Start

Begin by lying on the back. You can walk around the room and gently lift the students' arms or legs and rock them side to side, or the students can pair up and take turns performing this exercise. The arms or legs should be very relaxed and heavy, like overcooked macaroni—all soft and floppy.

MELTDOWN

▪ **Relaxation**

This relaxation exercise can also be interspersed within the yoga class to help students relax after challenging poses.

Start

Begin in any relaxation pose, with the eyes closed and the focus on the breath becoming relaxed.

PART 1

Slowly count back from 5 to 1 on each of your exhales. Tell students that with each exhale, they will gradually relax more and more. Give the following instructions and cues:

1. Let's focus on the lower body. Exhale 5 and relax; exhale 4 and relax your lower body even more; exhale 3 and relax your legs; exhale 2 and make your lower body still and quiet; and finally, exhale 1 and your whole lower body is relaxed.

2. Now we will focus on the core of the body, from the hips to the top of the shoulders.

3. Exhale 5 and relax; exhale 4 and relax your heart space even more; exhale 3 and relax your belly; exhale 2 and make your arms and hands still and quiet; and finally, exhale 1 and your whole lower body and core are relaxed.

4. We will focus on the neck and head now. Exhale 5 and relax; exhale 4 and relax your neck even more; exhale 3 and relax your skull; exhale 2 and make your face still and quiet; and finally, exhale 1 and your whole lower body is relaxed.

PART 2

Ask the students to take a few moments to become self-aware—where are they tight or holding stress? Tell them to take five more relaxed exhales to smooth and soothe any part of the body where they are holding onto stress.

PART 3

Cue the students by saying, "Sink into a deep relaxation. Slowly withdraw from the muscles, bones, and skin and sink deep within, listening to the quiet."

NOSE TO KNEES

(can also be called hugs or bug in a rug)

▪ **Relaxation**

Nose to knees pose helps the students relax their backs and helps with digestion as well.

Start

Begin by lying on the back.

1. Bend the knees, and keep the feet flat on the floor (this is called hook line position; see figure 6.10).

2. Inhale while bringing both arms over the head, and reach the fingertips to the wall behind you, touching the back of the hands on the floor.

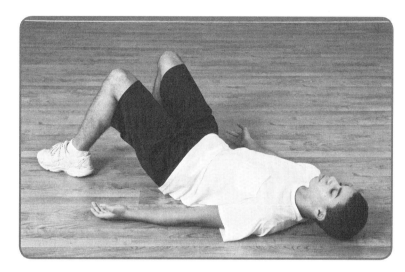

FIGURE 6.10 Hook line position.

3. Exhale and bring the arms to the chest while bending one knee. Use your arms to gently guide the knee to the chest to give it a hug. The head can remain on the ground, or you can lift the head, with the chin tucked into the chest.

4. Inhale and release the foot back to the ground, moving the arms back overhead.

5. Repeat on the other side.

6. Bring both knees in and hug them, coming into nose to knees (see figure 6.11).

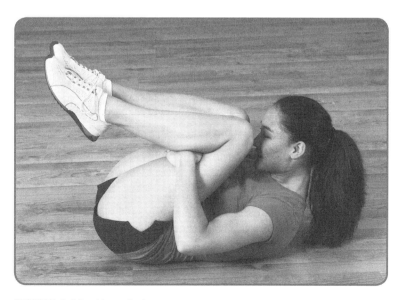

FIGURE 6.11 Nose to knees.

RELAXATION POSE

(Can also be called Shavasana, quiet pose, or Sleeping Beauty)

▪ Relaxation

Traditionally, the final relaxation pose in yoga is called Shavasana (see figure 6.12). In Sanskrit, *shavasana* means corpse.

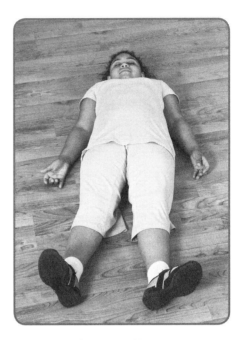

FIGURE 6.12 Relaxation pose.

1. If you feel comfortable, gently close your eyes or relax your eyes with a soft gaze forward. Imagine you can look down on your body and see it relaxed and rested. Allow your face to relax.

2. Extend and stretch out the legs, and let them gently move side to side. Relax the legs, allowing the toes to turn out to the sides, with the feet about 10 inches (25 centimeters) apart.

3. Lengthen the back, letting the arms rest comfortably, 5-7 inches (13-18 centimeters) from the side of the body with the palms facing upward, fingers relaxed and in the shape of an "A."

4. Turn the head gently side to side, and then release it so the back of the head is comfortably resting on the floor.

5. Say to the students, "Invite your eyes to close and the face to relax."

6. We are going to scan or check our bodies. Starting at the toes, picture in your mind each part of the body as I say it. You can also say quietly to yourself, "My feet are heavy" or *relaxed, soft, melting, quiet,* or *peaceful*—use whatever word sounds right to you.

7. Let the breath be slow, easy, and smooth.

8. Gently shifting your attention, bring your awareness to your legs. Say gently to yourself, "My legs are very heavy," and imagine your legs like jelly with no bones and the muscles very soft and relaxed.

   ▶ Continue through each of the body parts, pausing after each instruction and observing to see what students are doing.

9. Slowly start to come back from your relaxation time to this yoga space. Quietly, without the person next to you hearing you, slowly wiggle your fingers and toes. Slowly open your eyes, and rest your eye gaze in front of you for a moment.

10. Let's come into superstretch. Superstretch is when you reach your fingers up and over your head to the wall behind you, with your toes pointing in the opposite direction, reaching for the wall in front of you or the center of the circle. [pause] See if there is any other stretch your body needs to feel balanced and ready for our next activity.

11. Slowly curl up onto your side in fetal pose, and rest there with deep, full breaths.

> ▶ At this time, a short reflection can be done. For example, ask students to think about the yoga lesson's theme on friendship or how we are all teachers and how much we like to learn and teach.

12. Slowly roll up, and come into cross-legged seated pose. Let's take a few minutes before we end class to just enjoy breathing.

The purpose of relaxation or quiet time is not to fall asleep but to become relaxed in a mindful and attentive manner. Sometimes a student might fall asleep and snore, and this can be embarrassing. Keep your attention on students' body language and sounds. If you notice a student falling asleep, gently tap him on the arm with a soothing voice of assurance that everything is okay and to just relax.

Also included in this section are scripts to guide progressive muscle relaxation (PMR) and autogenic training. Both of these exercises are common methods used for stress management. The distinction between the two is, PMR helps students recognize muscle tension in various areas of the body and then how to relax those areas. Autogenic training means to self-generate relaxation or train the body and mind to be open to self-suggestion. The students focus on a body part, and without moving the body part, say to themselves that it is relaxed (e.g., "My hand is warm and relaxed. My hand is warm and relaxed"). You can offer words to encourage this process, but students are encouraged to use words that are meaningful and help them relax.

VOLCANO

■ **Relaxation**

Volcano is a progressive muscle relaxation exercise. PMR exercises allow the students to feel tension and then release it, just like a volcano that builds up heat and then lets it go.

Start

Begin in any relaxation pose, with the eyes closed and the focus on the breath becoming relaxed.

1. Point the toes as far as you can, and hold this position. With the next exhale, release the tension and wiggle the toes. Imagine the feet warm and relaxed like molten lava.

2. Lift your legs 2-3 inches (5-8 centimeters) from the ground—make all the muscles in the legs hard, hold it, and now let them relax into the floor like cooked noodles.

3. Tighten the gluteal muscles and hold. Now release the gluteals, and let them melt into the floor underneath.

4. Tighten the belly muscles and hold. Now let them relax. Take a long, relaxing breath and let it out very slowly. Allow the entire belly area to become soft and warm.

5. Clench the fists and make "arms of steel." Hold and then relax.

6. Pull the shoulders up to the ears—really shrug them. Hold this position, and now take a big sigh and release and relax the shoulders.

7. Bring the chin into the chest, hold it, and then relax the head back and gently turn the head side to side. Bring the head back and take a deep, relaxing breath.

8. Say to the students, "Scrunch up your face as if you ate a sour pickle or a lemon, hold it, and now relax your face. Let there be no muscles in your face, as if your face muscles have melted. Take a few more deep, relaxing breaths, and enjoy your whole body feeling very relaxed—feel your body flowing like molten lava."

Visualization and Guided Imagination

The relaxation exercises can also be made richer and tap into multiple intelligences by using visualization. Visualization provides cues that help students focus on what the pose or exercise might look like. Guided imagination takes visualization a step further by providing cues that are multisensory and appeal to different learning styles by using the various senses. Guided imagination is not about forcing thoughts or images on the students but allows for the students to use their own imagination and creativity. You can also add content from readings and poems students are studying.

The beauty of guided imagination is it lets you, the instructor, be creative by writing personal scripts or substituting words or images into existing scripts that might be useful for your specific students. Students can also be asked to write their own scripts as a creative writing project and start a collection of favorite relaxation scripts. A fun way to incorporate karma yoga (service to others) is to make a recording of these scripts and sell them, with the proceeds donated to a favorite charity.

COLOR ME PEACEFUL

▪ **Visualization**

This exercise brings the element of students imagining their favorite colors washing over their bodies, making them feel relaxed.

Start

Ask students to pick a favorite color, and imagine with each breath that beautiful favorite color filling up the whole body and making it feel warm and very comfortable.

Infusion Idea

The students can draw a picture of themselves in relaxation pose and color it with their favorite colors. Students can put the pictures in a special place to remind them that all they have to do is picture themselves in this pose to feel relaxed.

PUFFY CLOUDS

▨ **Visualization**

This exercise allows the students to imagine themselves relaxing on a gentle cloud. The following is a sample visualization script.

Start

1. Imagine you are resting in relaxation pose, not on the floor but on a big, fluffy, white cloud. Your whole body floats without any effort or weight.
2. Become as comfortable and relaxed as possible as you sink into this wonderful, soft, white, puffy cloud.
3. Pretend you are slowly rising up on your fluffy cloud and drifting on a gentle breeze in the blue sky, letting your breath be relaxed and soft.

STAR LIGHT, STAR BRIGHT

▨ **Visualization**

This exercise allows the students to imagine a beautiful star up in the sky. Begin by lying on the floor with the feet about 2 feet (0.6 meter) apart, arms in airplane with palms up. The following is a sample visualization script.

Start

1. We can do the star pose while standing, but we can also think about a shining star when we are relaxing. Think of your body as a beautiful star: brilliant and shining in the sky. Sprinkle your head with stardust. Now, sprinkle your arms, your core, and your legs—all with sparkling stardust.
2. There is beautiful stardust sprinkled all over you, and you feel bright and shiny but relaxed and peaceful.

STARFISH

▨ **Visualization**

This exercise allows the students to imagine being deep down on the ocean floor, resting quietly like a starfish. The following is a sample visualization script.

Start

1. Imagine you are a starfish resting deep down at the bottom of the ocean. It is very quiet, still, and peaceful here.
2. Allow your body to find whatever shape is best to feel completely relaxed as you float over the relaxing and soft sand.
3. Take a few more breaths as you become even more relaxed.

A SPECIAL MEADOW

■ **Guided Imagination**

With practice, instructors can easily come up with creative scripts that can link to any important topic or theme. A creative writing exercise is to ask students to write their own scripts and use them in class.

Start

Students are in their favorite relaxation poses. The following is a sample guided imagination script.

1. Gently close your eyes, and take in a few deep and relaxing breaths.
2. Imagine you are relaxing comfortably in a huge meadow.
3. Allow your breath to become as relaxed and quiet as possible.
4. Notice the blue sky with puffy, cotton-white clouds.
5. Smell the fresh and clean air.
6. Listen to the birds singing and the sharp cry of a blue jay calling for his friends.
7. Watch yourself as you walk over the green field full of vibrantly colored flowers.
8. Feel the grass, which is slightly wet against your legs, as it tickles your toes.
9. Inhale the scent of the wildflowers.
10. Enjoy the relaxing, and soak in all the beauty of the natural surroundings of this wonderful place through your imagination of taste, touch, sound, smell, and sight.
11. Come back slowly from your gorgeous meadow to this room by slowly stretching.
12. Slowly open your eyes, and let your gaze rest gently in front of you for a moment.

USING AN AUTOGENIC RELAXATION SCRIPT: THE WARM FUZZIES SCRIPT

■ **Guided Imagination**

Autogenics means self-creating, meaning the students are creating the feeling of relaxation by suggesting to themselves their bodies are warm and relaxed. This exercise sounds as if it might be easier for older students, but the younger students also enjoy the creativity of this exercise.

Start

This activity can be done lying down or sitting in a chair. The following is a sample guided imagination script.

1. Get as comfortable as possible. Gently close your eyes, and take a nice long breath through your nose; slowly exhale through your nose. Try a few more deep, relaxing breaths.

2. Bring your attention to your arms and hands. Feel them gently supported by the floor [or desk] below. Breathing slowly and without moving, say silently to yourself, *My arms and hands are heavy.* Say this three more times to yourself.

3. Bring your attention to your legs and feet. Be aware of the thigh, knee, lower leg, ankle, foot, and toes. Breathing slowly and without moving, say silently to yourself, *My legs are heavy.* Say this three more times to yourself.

4. Bring your attention to your arms again, and say silently to yourself, *My arms are warm.* Say this three more times to yourself.

5. Bring your attention to your legs again, and say silently to yourself, *My legs are warm.* Say this three more times to yourself.

6. Bring your attention to your arms and legs. Notice how they feel—very heavy and warm.

7. Now let your attention move to your entire body. Feel the spreading of heaviness and warmth to your arms, neck, shoulders, heart, belly, and legs. Take a deep breath, and say silently to yourself, *My whole body feels warm and heavy.* Repeat this three more times.

8. Notice how comfortable, quiet, and still the body feels. If you feel any tension, anywhere in your body, imagine feelings of warmth and heaviness spreading to that area.

9. Allow yourself to enjoy this feeling of deep relaxation by remaining still and quiet. Take three more deep, relaxing breaths.

10. As we say goodbye to our relaxation time together, gently start to wiggle your fingers and toes. Keeping your eyes closed, slowly come onto your side, and rest with your knees in toward your chest. Open your eyes slowly, and come up to a sitting position. Take a few more deep breaths before we end.

Meditation

As discussed in chapter 2, meditation is an integral part of yoga practice. Often the word conjures pictures of people sitting in lotus position (one leg crossed up over the other leg like a human pretzel) with the eyes closed in some blissful state, chanting weird-sounding noises. Students will often mimic this picture when the words *yoga* or *meditation* are mentioned.

Yoga poses and breath exercises were originally practiced to better facilitate sitting for long periods of time in meditation. Sitting quietly and looking at a candle flame, repeating a word, saying a prayer, thinking about an intention or a phrase, listening to music or a poem, or listening to one's own breath are all examples of ways to meditate. Research on the benefits of meditation is beginning to show it to be a strong tool anyone can use to become more focused, alert, mindful, and relaxed. The term *reflection time* might better convey the purpose of meditation and how it can be used with your students. Often in the busy and hurried world, there is little time devoted to inward reflection. Good teaching allows students to understand content as well as its application toward their lives. Reflection allows for this process to happen.

There are many creative ways to include meditation or reflection time in yoga class. Reflection time does not need to be at the end of class; it can also be included at the beginning of class, when students might choose an intention for their practice such as "I will be calm and strong in yoga today" and then reflect back on this intention at the end of class. Reflection can also involve asking students to reflect for a minute on being grateful or to silently thank all the teachers they have had in their lives. Reflection can be facilitated not only by quiet sitting or lying still but also by writing or drawing.

Meditation can also be cultivated by repeating a word silently over and over, such as *peace*, *shalom*, or *ohm*. The word *ohm* is a universal sound signifying that in this universe, we are all one and are part of this universal sound. The word *home* could be used instead to evoke the idea of a place one feels welcomed and at peace. Students can write a positive affirming statement about themselves on an index card and repeat it over and over again, such as "I am relaxed. I am strong. I am a good friend." Meditation can be as simple as observing the breath and, when the mind gets distracted, allowing the focus to come back to whatever aspect of the breath helps keep one anchored, such as the feeling of the breath on the back of the throat or as it enters into the nose. Counting the breath is often used as a focus in meditation (e.g., gently counting four breaths and starting over again after becoming distracted or after reaching the count of four breaths). Meditation can also be done while focusing on an image such as a flower. Keeping copies of classic art in the classroom and having students quietly look at these images can be very soothing. Van Gogh's *Sunflowers* and Monet's *Water Lilies* are just two suggestions.

Meditation does not always need to be done while seated or lying still. A walking meditation can be used to get students moving and focused. An outdoor excursion to a nature trail could allow students to meditate on all the colors they notice in the woods or to specifically notice all the different shades of green they encounter. A walking meditation can be done in the yoga class by having students move slowly and deliberately without touching anyone. Encourage this meditation by asking students to notice how their bodies move when walking, bringing the focus to the feeling of the feet making contact with the ground, the shifting of weight, the muscles used, and how the upper body helps with walking.

SUMMARY

When the relaxation time is finished, a final ending ritual to the class can be done. A poem can be read, for example. Traditionally at the end of yoga class, participants bow forward and say the Sanskrit word *namaste*, pronounced na-ma-stay. This word has several interpretations, but it means "May the energy, light, divine within me honor the energy, light, divine within you." Teaching yoga to children can be such a wonderful experience because after each class you may notice that you have received much more back from your students than you could have ever given them! This is the gift of yoga.

I honor the place in you where the universe resides. I honor the place in you of light, of love, and of truth.

I honor that place, and when you are in that place in you and I am in that place in me, we are one. Namaste.

chapter 7

Warm-Up, Active, and Cool-Down Poses

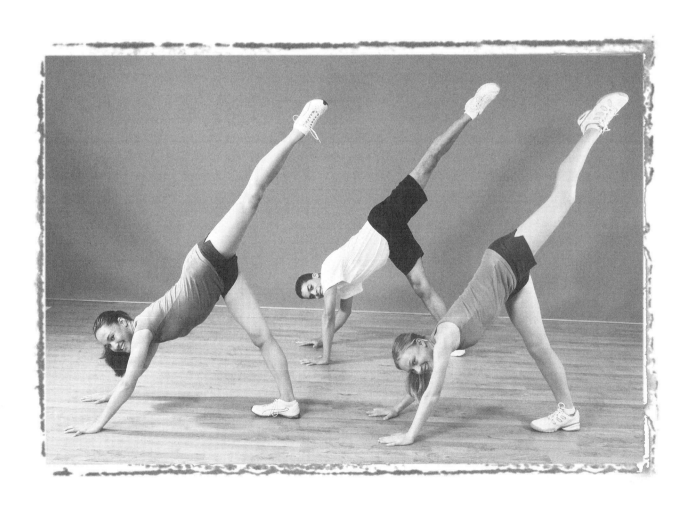

*T*here are hundreds of yoga poses, or asanas, pronounced ah-san-nas. The asanas selected for this book are basic, with safety being of utmost concern. The word *asana* means to hold steady and comfortable. In yoga, growth occurs by challenging the body and mind, but comfort and safety should always be the chief concern.

This chapter includes steps for introducing each pose and activity as well as steps for teaching correct alignment, or form. The warm-up poses help gently warm up and wake up the body and connect the breath to the body's movement. The active standing, moving, balancing, and floor poses are practiced in order to strengthen muscles, ligaments, tendons, and nerves. These poses also benefit the organs and endocrine glands as well as the brain cells. Poses that allow the spine to spiral help stretch the connective tissue of the back bones (vertebrae), decrease compression of the discs, and stimulate the spinal nerves. In addition, spinal spirals tone and massage the organs and glands and relieve tension in the back and hip areas. The final section includes cool-down poses that allow the body to further feel the benefits of stretching and can also be interspersed between more-active poses to bring balance to the body and mind.

WARM UP AND WAKE UP

Warm-up poses and exercises do just that—they wake up both the body and mind for the yoga practice. Warm-up exercises are done in a way that links the breath with simple movement. Linking the breath with movement allows students to connect how the breath is part of movement and not separate; the body and breath move as a unit, an integrative whole. If the breath is practiced with the body's movement over and over again, this natural way of moving becomes intuitive.

Warm-Up Exercises on the Floor

After beginning class with a breathing exercise or class opening ritual, warm-up poses linked with the breath slowly prepare the body and mind for yoga practice.

COBRA

(can also be called snake)

▦ **Warm-Up**

The cobra is a core strengthener. You will notice that infants do the cobra in order to gain enough core strength to be able to start creeping and crawling. In cobra, the hands are not doing the work but are used more for balance. The work comes from a strong foundation of an engaged core (see figure 7.1).

Pre-K+

Set up the exercise by saying, "Snakes can climb trees with no arms or legs. Can you? Snakes use their spines to move."

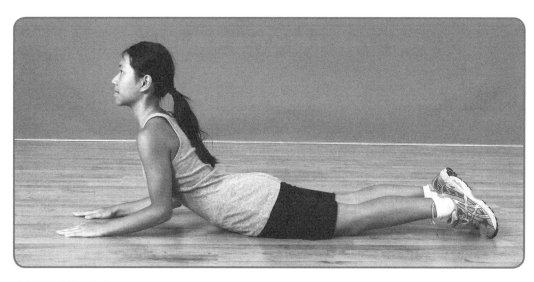

FIGURE 7.1   Cobra pose.

1. Start prone on the belly, and bring the legs together like the long tail of a snake.
2. Place the hands at the chest line, right under the shoulders, fingers pointed forward with the elbows bent and kept close to the sides of the ribs.
3. Press the hands into the floor and gently lift the chest, with the head in line with the spine (not extended back). Feel the length in the back.
4. Keep the lower body strong and grounded into the floor; keep the back fluid, and open the front of the body.

Pre-K-2

Ask the students to stick out their tongues and make a sound like a snake.

Grades 3+

Tell the class, "Press the heart forward as you 'shed' your skin behind you."

Infusion Idea

High school and older: "What mistakes have you made in the past that you can let go of and leave behind so that you can move forward?"

DOWNWARD-FACING DOG

(can also be called down dog, upside-down V, or inverted V)

■ **Warm-Up**

Downward-facing dog is a pose that at first may not seem relaxing, but as the students become familiar with it, they will love hanging out in the down dog! When teaching the down dog, ask the students to imagine themselves as an upside down V. Students tend to do the down dog like a push-up, with all their weight over their

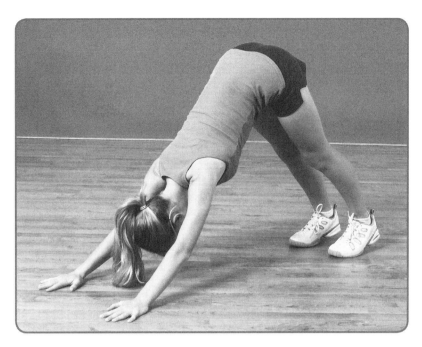

FIGURE 7.2 Downward-facing dog.

arms and wrists, rather than pressing their hips up to the sky and pressing their heart space back toward their legs (see figure 7.2). Encourage students to keep their hands spread wide and firmly planted into the ground and to stretch back.

Pre-K-2

Cue the students by saying, "From all fours [table pose], make the hands as large as big dog paws by planting them firmly on the mat, and lift your happy tail up to the sky. Bark like a happy puppy, ready to play!"

Grades 3+

From table pose

1. Place the hands flat on the floor straight ahead, fingers spread wide and strong.
2. Tuck the toes under and balance on the balls of the feet, keeping the feet hip-distance apart.
3. Straighten the legs and lift the hips up into an upside-down V shape—lift gluteals high and back (keep a dog tilt). The heels do not need to touch the ground.
4. Relax the head, and looking toward the knees, press the chest back toward strong legs.
5. Gently release this pose by bending both knees and coming back into table pose, then sit back into child pose.

Infusion Idea

Say to the class, "Have you noticed that lots of animals like to stretch? What kind of animals like to stretch? Can you show me? Animals know it is important to get exercise, to rest, and to stretch so they can be healthy and happy—we can learn a lot from them."

Variation A: Three-Legged Dog

Raise one arm or leg up in the air and balance on three "legs."

Variation B: Walk the Dog

Alternate bending one knee in toward the chest while pressing the other heel to the ground.

Variation C: Let's Go for a W-A-L-K

Move around the room in down dog.

GROWING CHILD

▪ Warm-Up

This warm-up exercise can help the students move from a quieting pose (child) to an opening and energizing pose (growing child). This pose helps the students lengthen and open up their spines so all the bones and muscles of the spine get a great stretch (see figure 7.3).

Start

1. From child, stretch the arms to the front, touching the floor in front of the body.

2. Inhale and come up to kneeling while sweeping the arms overhead and slightly back of the ears to get a long stretch throughout the spine, with a slight back bend. The eye gaze can be up at the arms overhead or looking straight ahead.

3. Take a few breaths while on the knees, and keep reaching with the arms. Then on the exhale, slowly move back into child and rest there.

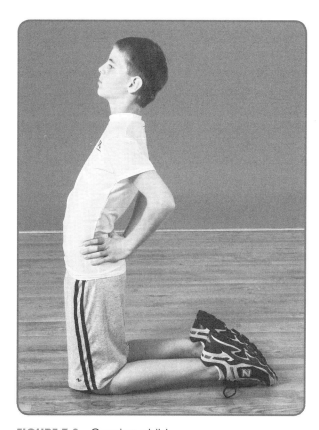

FIGURE 7.3 Growing child.

Variation

Tell students to place their hands on the small of their backs to help emphasize keeping the spine long and not collapsing the lower back.

ROCK THE BABY

Warm-Up

This pose allows the hips to be opened, but remind students to *gently* rock the baby (see figure 7.4).

Start

Begin in a cross-legged seated pose.

1. Lift one bent leg and hold underneath the knee with one hand and underneath the ankle with the other hand. Gently rock the knee side to side to open the hip joint, as if rocking a baby. Switch legs.

2. Finish in a cross-legged seated pose.

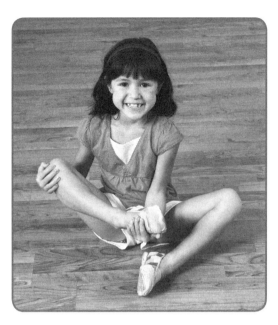

FIGURE 7.4 Rock the baby.

TABLE WITH COW AND CAT

Warm-Up

Table teaches good alignment and balance. It is a staple of most physical therapy exercises because it helps strengthen the core muscles (all the muscles of the torso, both front and back). This exercise helps students become familiar with the alignment and movement of their spines and especially of the tailbone. When we refer to the tailbone, we refer to its tilt, or the direction the tailbone is pointing, which is pivotal in the alignment of the spine. In table, the tailbone is in neutral, pointing straight back. When the tailbone is lifted up, this is called *dog tilt*, like a dog raising its tail up when it is happy to see you. Conversely, when the tailbone is tucked down and under, this is called *cat tilt*. The tailbone is tucked between the sit bones by drawing the belly button to the spine, like when a cat or dog is scared. By helping students feel the difference between these two tilts, they will be better able to replicate the tilts when in other poses (see figure 7.5, *a* through *c*).

Start

1. Table: Come onto all fours (on knees and palms of hands). Make sure the hands are flat and spread wide and the body weight is distributed evenly over the wrists, hands, and knees (see figure 7.5*a*). Let students know that if their wrists bother them, they can use fists instead of flat hands.

   - The hands are shoulder-width apart, with the shoulders directly over the wrists.

   - The knees are hip-width apart, with the toes pointed to the back; engage the core muscles to keep the back straight.

2. Cow: On the inhale, slowly raise the head and let the back sag, or sway, and the tailbone rise (see figure 7.5b).

3. Cat: On the exhale, rise up and arch the back like a scared cat. Let the head drop, bringing the chin toward the chest, and tuck the tailbone down and under (see figure 7.5c). Finish by sitting back on the heels and lowering the chest to the thighs in child pose. Come back to table.

4. Table: Cue the students by saying, "Your back should be strong and straight so I can put a bowl of soup on it."

Variation A, Pre-K+: Cricket Dancing

Begin in the table pose.

1. On the exhale, bend one knee into the chest. Drop the head, round the back, and touch the forehead close to the bent knee (see figure 7.6).

2. Inhale and extend the leg back to horizontal, lifting the head and chest. Avoid lifting the leg too high, which will cause too much of an arch in the back.

3. Return to table and switch sides.

Variation B, Pre-K+: Sneaky Cat

Begin in the table pose.

1. Inhale and reach the right arm forward to horizontal. Hold. Keep the back straight and strong. On the next exhale, return to all fours. Tell the students they can let their fingers spread wide and curl like a cat's paw.

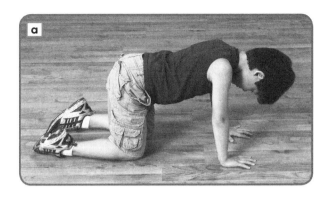

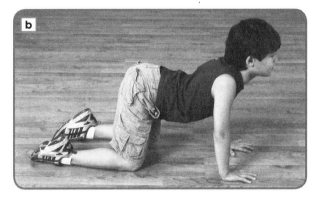

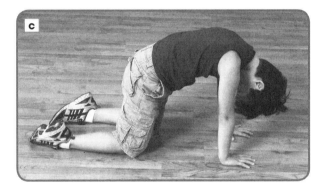

FIGURE 7.5 *(a)* Table pose, *(b)* cow pose, and *(c)* cat pose.

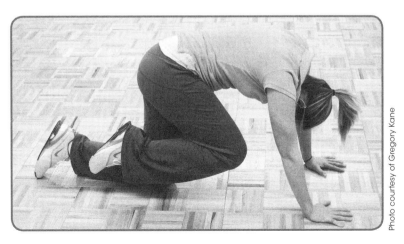

FIGURE 7.6 Cricket dancing.

2. Inhale and reach the left leg back to horizontal. Hold. On the next exhale, return to all fours.

3. Repeat, alternating each side to move slowly forward like a cat quietly sneaking up on a squeaky toy.

Variation C: Grade 3+ Balancing Table

Begin in the table pose.

1. Inhale and slide the right arm forward. Raise it and hold it at shoulder height; at the same time, let the left leg stretch back, raise it to horizontal, and balance (see figure 7.7). Keep the eye gaze on a focus point. Keep the core of the body strong without tilting. Ask the students to imagine a cup of water on the table (the back). Tell them not to let any water spill. Hold this balance for a few breaths, and then return to table.

2. Repeat with the left arm and right leg. It will take the students some time to coordinate the opposite limbs moving.

3. Finish by returning to table, then sit back into child.

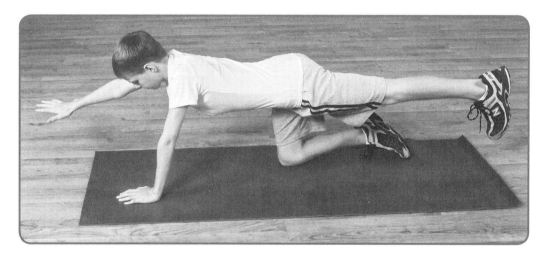

FIGURE 7.7 Balancing table.

TURNING TOPS

▪ Warm-Up

This movement exercise pairs the breath with spiraling movements of the spine (see figure 7.8), allowing the students to move the spine in several directions, which is useful after sitting in one position for a while, such as staring at a computer screen.

Start

Begin in a cross-legged seated pose, hands resting on thighs.

1. Inhale, sweep the arms out to the sides, and reach up overhead.

2. Exhale and bring the hands back to the thighs.

3. Again, inhale and sit tall, with arms sweeping out and up.

4. Exhale and spiral to the right by turning the belly button to the right, reaching the left hand to rest on the right thigh. Reach the right arm around to the right to deepen the twist. Take a deep breath.

5. On the next inhale, slowly bring both arms back overhead; on the next exhale, spiral to the left by turning the belly button to the left.

6. Take a deep inhalation, and return to start.

▶ In spiraling movements, which are spine twists, emphasize moving from the core, the movement starting with the turning of the belly button. This discourages twisting from the upper spine first and overstressing the neck or shoulders.

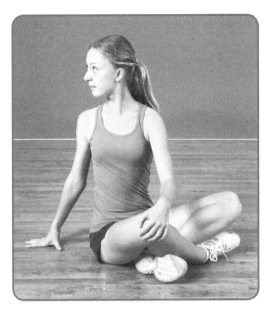

FIGURE 7.8 Turning tops.

UPWARD-FACING DOG

(can also be called up dog)

■ **Warm-Up**

Upward-facing dog is the counterpose that balances the downward-facing dog. You will notice that animals naturally move from downward-facing dog into upward-facing dog. Encourage students to keep their upper bodies strong with the core engaged, not allowing the shoulders to collapse but keeping the shoulder blades down and the heart lifted (see figure 7.9).

Pre-K+

From downward-facing dog, stretch forward onto the toes and hands. Tell students to make a big, happy puppy grin. Move back and forth from downward-facing dog to upward-facing dog a few times, and then rest in child pose. Finish in table or child.

Grades 3+

From downward-facing dog and without moving the hands and feet, drop the back and legs down, keeping the legs firm and strong while looking

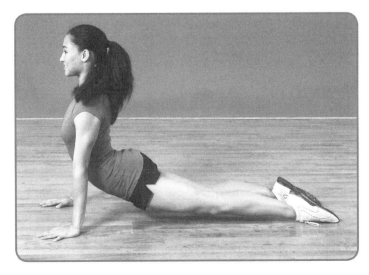

FIGURE 7.9 Upward-facing dog.

forward. The back will bow slightly, but keep the shoulders firm, chest lifted and strong, and avoid letting the shoulders drop and cave in. Hold while resting the tops of the feet (toes are pointed) and lower shins on the floor, or drop the knees to the floor. End in downward-facing dog or child.

YOGA JUMPING JACKS

■ **Warm-Up**

This exercise helps the students feel how the inhalation energizes and moves the body, while the exhalation brings the body back to relaxation.

Start

Begin lying flat on the back, with the arms alongside the body.

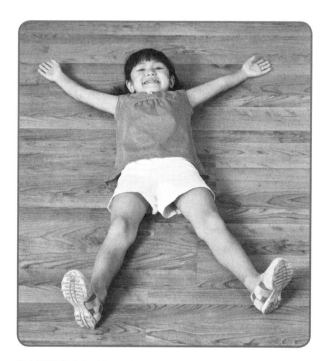

1. Take a moment to feel the body on the floor.

2. Slowly working from the feet to the top of the head, let the body feel even more relaxed as it melts into the supportive floor underneath with each exhale.

3. Pay attention and notice the points of contact the body makes, feeling the back of the legs, the arms, the backside, the shoulders, and the head resting gently on the floor.

FIGURE 7.10 Yoga jumping jacks.

4. Inhale and slowly raise the arms over the head, reaching the fingertips to the wall behind you, touching the back of the hands on the floor. Separate and move each leg out to the side like a jumping jack (see figure 7.10). Take another inhalation, and feel how strong and energized your body feels.

5. Exhale and slowly return the arms to the sides of the body and the legs together. Rest here for a moment.

6. Cue the students by saying, "We can pretend we are doing jumping jacks in a big swimming pool filled with mud or jelly, so we are going very slowly. Can you move even slower with your breath as you move out to jumping jack and back?"

Moving Warm-Up Exercises

After the warm-up exercise on the floor, take the students into a more-active warm-up with some shake it and wake it exercises. Especially with younger students (pre-K-2), starting a yoga class seated is not going to work on any given day (think of the saying "ants in their pants"!). What is described here may not sound like yoga, but it does sound like a creative outlet for your students to let off a little steam and get warmed up.

HEAVY BUCKET SWING

▪ **Moving Warm-Up**

This pose helps students use their imagination to allow their arms to swing freely as if holding buckets of cement.

Start

1. From standing, exhale. Bend the knees and reach the arms forward, telling the students to imagine they are holding two heavy buckets of sand or cement (see figure 7.11).

2. Inhale. Gently swing the buckets up overhead, and stand as tall as possible.

3. Exhale. Gently swing the buckets back to the ground and past the knees, making a big "ha" sound as the buckets swing down and drop. Repeat.

4. Drop the buckets. Bend forward and hug the bent knees while standing.

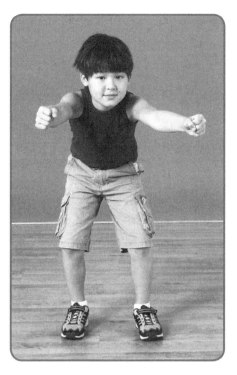

FIGURE 7.11 Heavy bucket swing.

SHAKE IT UP

▪ **Moving Warm-Up**

This moving series of poses allows the students to connect with and move with the entire body. Set up the exercise by saying, "Let's start from head to toe, waking up and shaking up!"

Start

Begin standing in the yoga space or on a mat.

1. Tell the children to use their noses to draw circles, their names, or big squiggly lines, as if a chalkboard is in front of their faces.

2. Start to move the shoulders up and down. Circle and roll the shoulders back for three circles, and now roll them to the front. Lift the shoulders high (right up to the ears), and let them drop down with a loud sigh. Swim forward with the elbows bent and the hands holding the shoulders, and now swim backward. Do the dog paddle.

3. Wiggle the hips and make big circles, as if you are using a hula hoop.

4. Tell the students to hop on one foot, balance, and write their names with the foot that's in the air. Switch.

5. Start swirling side to side with the arms at your sides like a plane propeller or cement mixer (see figure 7.12). Now stretch the arms straight out to the sides, strong in airplane arms. Bend forward at the hips and reach across and down with one hand to the opposite knee, while the other arm reaches and extends up to the sky. Now switch to the other side.

6. Say to the class, "Now, when I say *Go*, we are going to start moving around the room, but be careful to be respectful and mindful as you move and not touch anyone. You can hop, skip, leapfrog, jog, gallop, jump—any way you can move safely! When I say *Freeze*, find a mat or space and freeze into whatever yoga pose I say. Ready? Go!"

7. "Freeze! Hold the _____ pose, keep breathing, smile. OK, ready? Go! Let's move again."

Variation

Most of the movements in steps 1 and 2 of shake it up can be done in a chair.

Infusion Idea

Equipment such as soft (Nerf) balls, hoops, scooters, and scarves can be used during this general warm-up. Music or a drum can be used to signal students to begin movement and to stop and freeze.

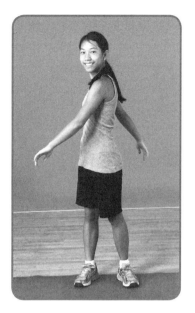

FIGURE 7.12 Shake it up.

SOAKING-WET DOG

◾ **Moving Warm-Up**

This is the best pose: imitating a dog shaking off water after getting out of the bathtub or swimming in the lake. It helps students learn to shake off tension they may still be holding in the body long after the pose is over.

Start

This exercise can be done standing or in table pose (see figure 7.13).

1. Start by moving the head side to side (not too hard).

2. Tell the students to pretend they have floppy puppy dog ears, and then shake and move the arms, tummy, legs, toes, all the way down to the tailbone, shaking all the water off.

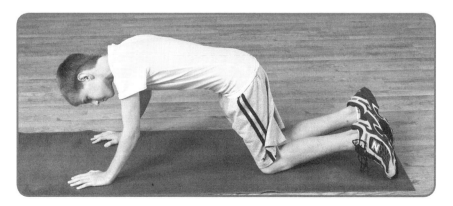

FIGURE 7.13 Soaking wet dog.

STANDING FROG INTO SQUAT

▪ **Moving Warm-Up**

This pose is a great stretch for the hip flexors. In yoga, this is often referred to as a "hip opener."

Start

1. Step out into a wide stance, and bend the knees into a squat with the knees over the ankles. Turn the right foot so it points to 2 o'clock and the left foot so it points to 10 o'clock. Bring the arms up, with the elbows bent at 90 degrees into "cactus arms." Hold, letting the tailbone, which is in neutral tilt, drop even further to the floor.

2. To allow for an even further stretch, place the hands or fingertips between the legs on the floor for balance, with elbows inside the knees (see figure 7.14).

3. Inhale. Squat as deeply as possible, lifting the head and chest. Tell the students to "catch a fly."

4. Exhale. Straighten the legs, come into wide-angle standing forward fold, and look between the legs.

5. Inhale. Repeat.

6. Slowly roll up the spine to standing.

Variation, Pre-K+

Leapfrog by moving around the room from a squat and jumping forward.

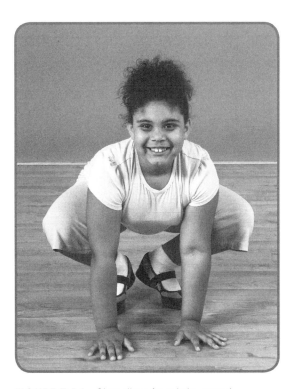

FIGURE 7.14 Standing frog into squat.

STANDING TWISTERS

(can also be called blenders)

▪ **Moving Warm-Up**

This pose helps students learn to move and keep their spines limber.

Start

Stand with the feet a little wider than hip-distance apart.

1. Keep the arms hanging loosely out at the sides of the body in a T shape—airplane arms (see figure 7.15).
2. Gently turn from the hips and swivel to one side; let the arms swing in the same direction and wrap around the body.
3. Gently come back to center, with arms in a T, and swing the other way.
4. Continue to swing back and forth, and slowly turn the head in the direction of the swing.

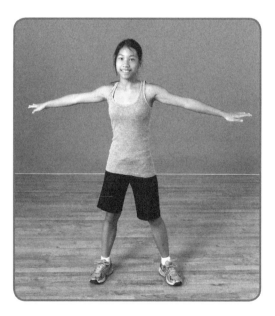

FIGURE 7.15 Standing twisters.

Variation, Pre-K+

Say to the class, "Think of a blender full of yummy fruit to make a smoothie—we want to make sure all the fruit gets mixed in!" Pre-K students will typically overswing into others or fall down, so make sure to contain the enthusiasm so no one gets hurt.

STANDING POSES

After the students have spent some time warming up, the next transition is to poses that help the students get stronger in their standing and postural muscles. However, you can teach a class that is done entirely seated with no standing for a variation or when the students might be tired. Standing poses help energize and wake up your students even more and help build strength and endurance. The importance of alignment and setting a foundation is discussed in chapter 4 and can be seen in figure 4.6 (page 57).

CHAIR

▪ **Standing Pose**

Chair is the speedskater's or skier's best friend as it encourages strength in the quadriceps and gluteals as well as engagement of a strong core (see figure 7.16).

Start

Begin in the mountain pose.

1. Place the feet hip-distance apart, keeping the feet and knees pointed straight ahead.

2. Sit down as if sitting in an imaginary chair; keep the knees bent, drop the gluteals down, and maintain the tailbone at a dog tilt. Keep weight back over the heels with the knees over the ankles.

3. Reach arms overhead and look at the hands.

4. Engage the core muscles, and lift the chest while relaxing the shoulders.

5. Finish in mountain.

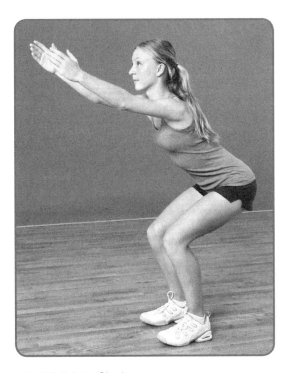

FIGURE 7.16 Chair.

CHEST STRETCHER

▪ **Standing Pose**

This pose helps with flexibility in the shoulders and helps open up the chest and heart space as well (see figure 7.17). Students will have a tendency to hold their arms up high, and as a result their shoulders become hunched—encourage the students to drop the clasped hands down to the midback or tailbone level and to keep the heart space open and lifted.

Start

Begin in mountain.

1. Standing tall, reach behind the back and clasp the hands or hold onto the wrist or elbow; lift gently, holding the hands at waist level.
2. Keep the shoulders and shoulder blades down, with an open chest.
3. Hinge at the hips, and come into standing forward fold while keeping the hands clasped. Hold.
4. Leading with the heart and with firm legs, slowly come back to mountain and release the hands.

Variation

Students can hold onto a yoga strap or towel if they cannot clasp their hands behind their backs.

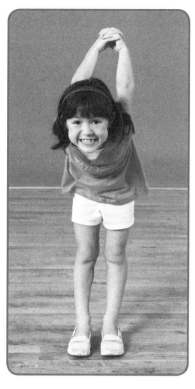

FIGURE 7.17 Chest stretcher.

ELEPHANT

▪ **Standing Pose**

This pose is a nice counterpose to balance chest stretcher. Begin in mountain, and then bring the hands together in front of the hips and clasp the wrists. Swing the arms side to side like an elephant trunk (see figure 7.18).

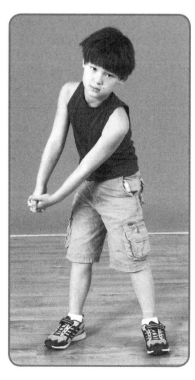

FIGURE 7.18 Elephant.

EXTENDED SIDE ANGLE

(can also be called super side stretch)

▪ **Standing Pose**

This pose engages everything—nothing is left behind, as the legs are engaged and strong and the top arm is reaching up and over the head (see figure 7.19).

Start

1. From warrior II with the right knee bent, bend the right arm and let the right forearm rest on the right bent knee, and extend the left arm up to sky, looking up at the hand. To advance, reach the left arm from over the head up and over to reach toward the right wall.

2. Keeping the left leg strong, press the left foot into the floor.

3. Press the legs firmly into the ground, and slowly come up and reverse.

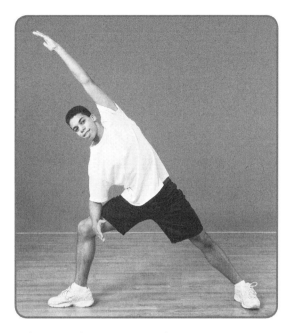

FIGURE 7.19 Extended side angle pose.

HALF MOON

▪ **Standing Pose**

Students love this pose because it is all about just going for it and saying any words of inspiration, such as "Yippee!" or "Yahoo!" or "_____!" (see figure 7.20).

Start

Begin from warrior II to the right.

1. Reach forward and to the side with the right hand, and balance on the fingertips while slowly extending the left leg. Reach up overhead with the left hand, and focus on the left fingertips.

2. Tell the students to say "Yahoo!" or whatever they feel like saying.

3. Bring the foot slowly to the ground, and slowly stand up.

4. Switch sides.

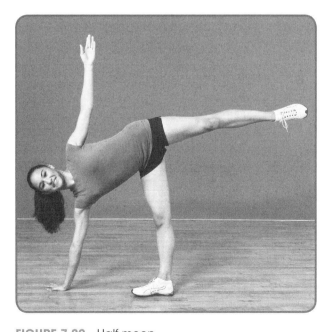

FIGURE 7.20 Half moon.

HORSE

■ **Standing Pose**

The horse is a fun way to introduce opposite-moving legs and arms. When the left leg comes up, the right arm goes up as well (see figure 7.21).

Start

Lift the left knee up to right-angle height or lower while simultaneously lifting the right arm up, elbow at right angle or lower and the hand shaped like a horse's hoof. Then switch with a hopping movement, letting the right arm and left leg drop and lifting the left arm and right knee up like a horse prancing.

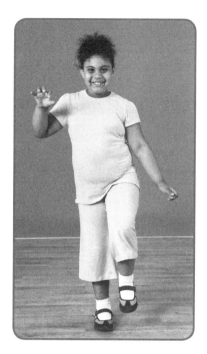

FIGURE 7.21 Horse.

MOUNTAIN

■ **Standing Pose**

Mountain is the pose from which most of the standing and balancing poses start (see figure 7.22). Reinforce with students the importance of setting the foundation and alignment of mountain. This pose should evoke feelings of quiet strength; the student feels strong but grounded and calm at the same time.

Start

Stand up straight with arms at the sides.

1. Keep the feet hip-distance apart, with toes and knees pointing straight ahead.
2. Keep the knees slightly bent (soft or relaxed).
3. Keep the legs, core muscles, and gluteals strong.
4. Keep the chest open and lifted; the arms can be brought overhead, reaching to the sky.

   ▶ Make sure to check the students' alignment.

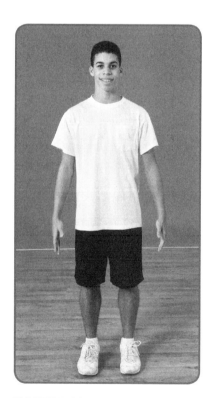

FIGURE 7.22 Mountain.

Variation

Students can stand with their backs to the wall and feel what it is like to stand up straight in mountain by feeling the back of the head, shoulder blades, gluteals, and heels against the wall.

Infusion Idea

For this "source of strength" exercise, cue the students by saying, "Think of the mountain pose as something solid that won't fall down. Now for a moment, think of what gives you strength. For example, family, friends, working hard, or eating healthy food. Feel the feet sinking deep into the ground and the crown of the head reaching toward the sky. Stand as strong and tall as you comfortably can."

You can go around the class and ask each student what gives her strength while she stands in mountain with her hands resting over her heart. If a student does not want to share, she can simply say, "Pass."

QUARTER MOON

(can also be called crescent moon, lateral flexion, or side bend)

▪ **Standing Pose**

Quarter moon is a lateral flexion movement, which is one of the four movements of the spine. It is critical to maintain a good level of lateral flexion throughout life in order to be able to move the spine with ease and freedom. Cue students to stay connected to their breath as they may have the tendency to overreach during the side bend, and their breath will subsequently become tight and jagged. It is also important to cue students to reach through both sides of the body like the shape of a crescent moon and not allow the bending side to collapse but to keep reaching out to the side wall and not down to the floor (see figure 7.23).

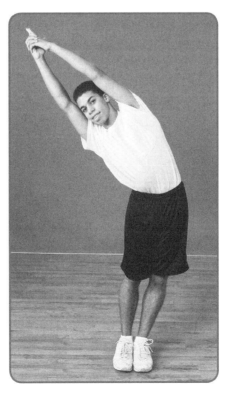

FIGURE 7.23 Quarter moon.

Start

Begin in mountain.

1. Extend the spine long and straight, keeping the core strong and the feet firmly planted on the ground throughout the pose.

2. Reach the arms overhead with hands clasped and index fingers pointed together, making a steeple.

3. Exhale. Stretch to the side, pointing the steeple to the side wall.

4. Remind students to check in with their breath to make sure it is full and deep and to find just the right amount of stretch. Tell them to ease off a bit if the breath becomes tight.

5. Inhale. Come back to arms overhead; keep the legs and feet firm.

6. Exhale. Repeat on the other side.

7. Finish in mountain with arms at the sides or hands folded over the heart.

Variation

With one hand, hold onto a sturdy chair that will not slip when there is weight put on it (it can be placed against the wall to prevent slipping). Reach the other arm up overhead, and reach to the side toward the chair.

ROCKET SHIP

■ **Standing Pose**

A nice counterpose after holding the chair pose, rocket ship allows the body to reach and stretch up to the sky (see figure 7.24).

Start

1. Squat down as far as possible in chair, keeping the feet and knees straight ahead.

2. Bring the hands in front of the chest in steeple position—hands clasped with index fingers pointed together.

3. Count 1, 2, 3 and shoot up into the air like a rocket, coming from chair and extending the legs to standing, arms reaching overhead with hands in steeple position.

4. Finish in mountain.

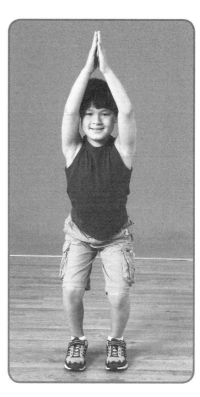

FIGURE 7.24 Rocket ship.

RUNNER'S LUNGE

▪ **Standing Pose**

Runner's lunge helps to strength the legs. Stretch the hips and challenge your students' balance and reinforce the knee alignment, centering over the ankle (see figure 7.25).

Start

Begin in the mountain pose.

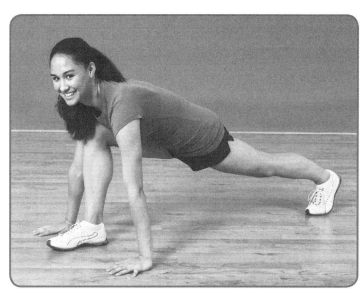

1. Come into standing forward fold, keeping the fingertips or flat palms on the floor, slightly in front of the feet.

FIGURE 7.25 Runner's lunge.

2. Step back firmly, keeping the left leg straight, and balance on the back left toes while the front right leg bends to 90 degrees. Keep the knee bent over the ankle, not over the toes.

3. Switch legs.

STANDING BACK BEND

(can also be called back extension)

▪ **Standing Pose**

This pose allows the front of the body to become open. Because our students spend a great deal of time with their spines flexed forward and the shoulders slouched, this pose helps them elongate and stretch out their spines. Standing back bend can make participants feel anxious or vulnerable as the heart and throat open. As discussed earlier, a student has full permission to come out of the pose early.

Start

Begin in the mountain pose.

1. Make sure the feet are firmly planted to the floor, with strong legs and core muscles.

2. Make fists with both hands, reach the arms up and then back, and place the fists just below the waist close to the spine at the level of the kidneys.

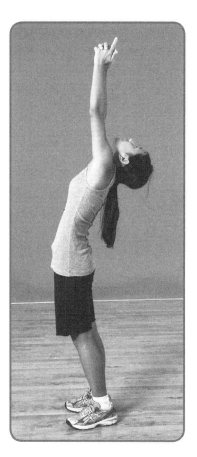

FIGURE 7.26 Standing back bend.

3. Pressing the fists into the lower back, bring the elbows close together behind the back, press the hips forward, and look up at the ceiling, feeling the chest and throat opening.

4. Keep the legs strong and the core engaged.

5. Remind students to check in with their breath. Tell them they can back off if it feels scary or the breath becomes tight. Students can also look forward if there is too much strain on the neck.

6. Finish in standing forward fold (see next pose).

Variation

Arms reach up overhead with hands together in steeple (see figure 7.26). Reach strong with fingers pointing up and back.

STANDING FORWARD FOLD

(can also be called rag doll or Jell-O melt)

▪ **Standing Pose**

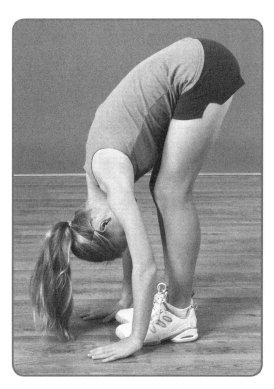

FIGURE 7.27 Standing forward fold.

The standing forward fold is relaxing because it is an inversion pose. The head is lower than the heart, allowing blood to flow to the brain instead of pumping against gravity when we are sitting or standing. This also allows the heart some relaxation in its never-ending workload of constantly pumping our blood. Sometimes, especially with older students, this pose becomes a contest to see who has the most flexibility, but emphasize that this is not a competition. Some students will have tight hamstrings, and this will be a challenging pose for them. Remind students to hang with no effort, to keep the knees slightly bent or even bend them more to take the strain off the hamstrings, to let the upper body feel loose and heavy, and to keep the neck relaxed and the eye gaze between the legs (see figure 7.27).

Start

Begin in the mountain pose.

1. Lift both arms to the sky.

2. Forward dive by hinging at the hips, keeping the back long and strong while reaching the arms forward and then down to the floor.

3. Let the arms and head hang down. Gently shake the head side to side so the neck is released.

4. Keep the knees bent so they are soft, or relaxed.

5. Hold onto each elbow, hold onto the legs or ankles, or just let the arms hang like a rag doll.

6. Gently bend the knees even more, and gently roll up the spine, with the head coming up last.

Variation

The forward fold does not need to be kept static; the students can explore gently swaying side to side or other micro (very small) movements, but avoid any bouncing or ballistic kinds of movement.

Infusion Idea

Pre-K students can sing "The itsy bitsy spider climbed up the water spout" as they gently come up, "Down came the rain" while falling forward into forward fold, and so on.

STANDING WIDE-ANGLE FORWARD FOLD

▪ **Standing Pose**

This standing wide-angle forward fold is also an inversion pose and challenges the hamstrings to lengthen (see figure 7.28).

Start

Begin in the mountain pose, and ask students to jump their feet out to the sides and keep the feet planted wide, with toes pointed straight ahead (wide-leg stance).

1. Reach up to the sky with the arms, then forward dive with a long spine and hinge at the hips.

2. Place the palms or fingertips in line with the feet on the floor, with knees as bent as necessary. The hands can also be placed anywhere on the legs.

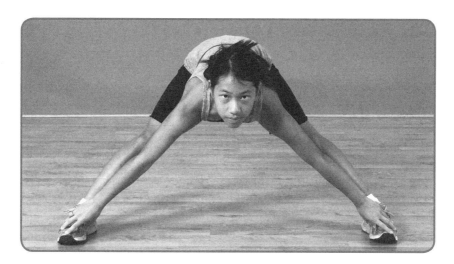

FIGURE 7.28 Standing wide-angle forward fold pose.

3. With legs strong, slowly reverse forward dive back to tall spine and jump legs together into standing.

Variation

Place a chair an arm's length away in front. Hinge at the hips and reach forward, with both hands holding onto the back of the chair or the seat of the chair for a deeper stretch.

Infusion Idea

A geometry lesson can be infused here by demonstrating that the wider the base of the triangle (i.e., the farther the feet are apart), the easier the pose gets.

TIPPING STAR

▪ **Standing Pose**

Tipping star (see figure 7.29) is a variation on lateral flexion. Ask students to keep the star in one plane. This means they don't reach forward to tip more but keep reaching to the side wall, keeping the whole body including the core in one plane and discouraging any twisting.

Start

Start in mountain.

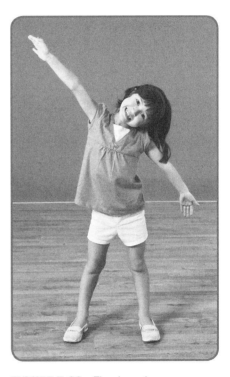

1. Jump out into a wide-leg stance, a little wider than hip-distance apart, with toes pointed straight ahead.

2. Bring the arms out to the sides, parallel to the ground, known as airplane arms.

3. Make the arms, legs, and neck strong like a five-point star.

FIGURE 7.29 Tipping star.

4. Exhale. Tip the star to the side.

5. Inhale. Stand tall again, and exhale and tip the star the other way.

TRIANGLE

▪ **Standing Pose**

In this pose, it is challenging to keep the legs strong and rooted into the ground (see figure 7.30).

Start

Begin in the mountain pose.

1. Jump out into a wide-leg stance about as far as one big walking step.

2. Turn one foot to point directly to the right and the other slightly to the right, with both legs staying strong and straight throughout the pose.

3. The hips and shoulders are square to the front, and the arms are straight over the legs at the sides (airplane arms).

4. Reach with the right arm to the side, hinge at the hip, reach out to the right side wall as far as possible, and then reach down to hold onto the shin or ankle. The left arm reaches up to the sky. Look up or at the floor.

5. Slowly come back up with strong legs and core, reverse the feet (point them to the left), and reach the left arm out to triangle on the left.

Variation

Set up chairs that students can hold onto as they reach out to the side.

Infusion Idea

Ask the students, "Where do we see triangles in our everyday life? How many triangles do our bodies make when we do triangle pose?"

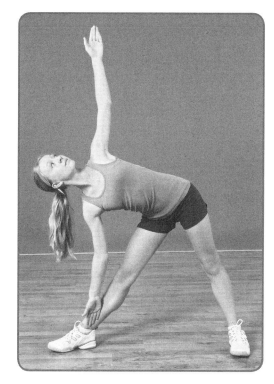

FIGURE 7.30 Triangle.

WARRIORS

▪ **Standing Pose**

The translation from Sanskrit of *warrior* is peacekeeper. There are three variations of warrior pose, and their purpose in yoga is to build strength—not for fighting or hurting others but the real strength needed to be a peacekeeper. Warrior I is done with the core and both feet facing forward. Warrior II is done with the core and the back foot facing to the side. Warrior III is warrior I tipped forward into the shape of a T (warrior III is described in the balancing poses section).

Pose: Warrior I

Warrior I is a total-body strengthening exercise: The legs hold the pose, the arms reach overhead, and the core is engaged to keep the pose steady and the spine strong (see figure 7.31*a*).

START

Begin in the mountain pose.

1. Take a big step back with the left foot into a lunge position, keeping the left leg firm and the left foot turned out slightly and grounded.

2. Keep the right foot straight ahead, with the knee bent over the ankle. (The right foot is at 12 o'clock, and the left foot is at 9 or 10 o'clock.)

3. Square the shoulders and hips to the front, with the core strong and lifted.

4. Reach overhead with both arms; keep a strong, straight back leg.

Variation: Kneeling Warrior

The front bent knee remains bent while the back knee is bent and placed on the floor for balance, the back toes flat on the ground. The upper body and arms remain reaching to the sky.

Infusion Idea

Say to the students, "The warriors in yoga are peacekeepers. How can we show we are peacekeepers?" Suggestions: using building statements instead of put-down statements and saying thank you.

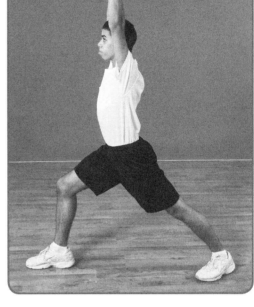

FIGURE 7.31a Warrior I.

Pose: Warrior II

Warrior II is an affirming pose for building self-confidence that students love (see figure 7.31b).

START

Begin in the mountain pose.

1. Jump into a wide-leg stance.

2. Turn both feet to face to the right. (The right foot is at 3 o'clock, and the left foot is at 12 o'clock.)

3. Bend the right knee over the right ankle, and keep the left leg strong and straight.

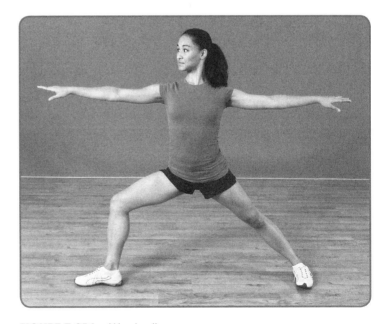

FIGURE 7.31b Warrior II.

4. Hold the arms in airplane, straight over the legs at the sides, and let the eye gaze look over the right fingertips.

5. Keep the shoulders and hips square to the side.

6. Maintain a slight cat tilt.

7. Return to a wide-leg stance, and reverse the feet to practice warrior II to the left.

Pose: Reverse Warrior

This pose allows for a modified side bend and opens up the ribs and chest (see figure 7.31c).

START

1. From warrior II to the right, drop the left arm to hold onto the straight left leg, and hold.

2. The right arm reaches to the sky and then reaches overhead to the left in a slight side bend. Keep the heart lifted and open. You can move from extended side angle (see page 123) to reverse warrior, moving like a teeter-totter. Return to a wide-leg stance, and reverse the feet to practice reverse warrior to the left.

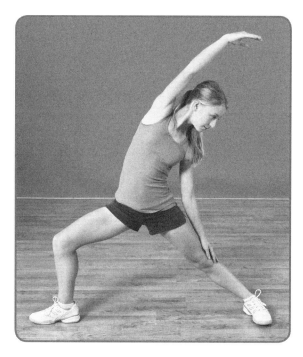

FIGURE 7.31c Reverse warrior.

MOVING YOGA

We now shift the focus and energy of the standing poses in a more dynamic and engaging way through what is called vinyasa, or moving yoga. A sun salutation is a series of successive yoga poses that are linked with the breath and emulate the cyclic movement of the sun and moon. There are traditional sun salutations with specific poses linked in a specific succession. However, the sun salutations presented here are offered as examples of opportunities to link various poses into movement. Both you and your students can invent fun and creative sun salutations. By using songs or music, the poses can have a theme that is integrated into the song or story. Put on some tunes and enjoy moving yoga (see the resources section for music ideas).

Students can make up sun salutations that mimic sports patterns or stories. Some of the new dance crazes such as the Cha Cha Slide can be infused with yoga poses, making them more fun. And students really come alive when pop music comes on board!

Here are some examples of sun salutations.

SILLY WIGGLE SUN DANCE

■ Moving Yoga, Pre-K-2

This sun salutation is a great way to link poses with some active wiggling and fun.

Start

Begin in the mountain pose.

1. Reach the arms up to the sky, then reach forward and walk on the hands and feet like a monkey.
2. Come into downward-facing dog—make the body like an upside-down V. Tell the students to wiggle their hips side to side like a puppy wagging his tail.
3. Lower your knees down into table, and make a big lion's roar.
4. Do balancing table to the right, come back to table, and now do balancing table to the left.
5. Come back to table and do soaking-wet dog pose. Shake all the water off!
6. Slowly come up into a squat, and wiggle side to side in squat position. Now jump forward like a leaping frog and come into standing forward fold—hug your knees and wiggle again. Slowly roll up your spine, and finish in mountain.

SUN DANCE

■ Moving Yoga

The sun dance is a simple sun salutation that allows for the series of connecting poses to be done in one spot.

Start

Start in child.

1. Move to table, and push up into downward-facing dog.
2. Move to table, and lower down into cobra.
3. From cobra, move back to table and then push back into downward-facing dog again.
4. After holding downward-facing dog for a few breaths, drop on the knees into table and sit back and rest in child to finish.

SUN, MOON, AND STAR DANCE

■ **Moving Yoga**

This sun salutation brings in more poses and is more active.

Start

Begin in mountain.

1. Jump out into a wide stance and do tipping star pose—tip the star to one side and then the other. Jump back to mountain.
2. Sit down into chair. Count 1, 2, 3 and rocket ship back up to the sun, to quarter moon pose to the right and quarter moon to the left, and finish in mountain.

Infusion Idea

Ask the students, "What would you take if you could take only one thing to the moon or the space station?"

SUNFLOWER AND CACTUS DANCE

■ **Moving Yoga**

This sun salutation emphasizes the creative movement of the arms (see figure 7.32).

Start

1. Stand with your feet wide apart, keeping your knees over the ankles in frog pose.
2. Bring the hands up into cactus arms (elbows held at shoulder level, with hands at right angles). While keeping the feet planted, start to move like a sunflower. Tell the class to reach and bend up to catch the rays of the sun.
3. Add music or a drum: Tell the students, "When the music stops, stop moving and come into the shape a sunflower might take when the sun goes away, but be still and strong."

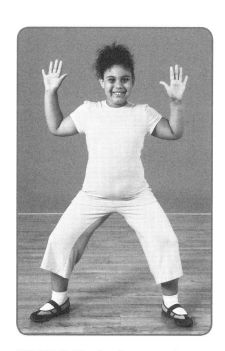

FIGURE 7.32 Sunflower and cactus dance.

BALANCING POSES

Learning to balance is a skill that needs to be practiced throughout the life span. It is an important component of daily activities and for sports as well. For your students, working on balance lays the foundation for a lifetime of good balancing mechanics to avoid the disastrous results of slipping and falling when they get older. Success at balancing poses can be aided by instructing students to keep a focus point, or dhristi. Finding a focus point will help students stay calm during these challenging balancing tasks.

ARROW

■ **Balancing Pose**

Arrow is a good all-body balancing and strengthening pose (see figure 7.33).

Start

Begin in warrior I.

1. Bend forward, bringing the chest over the front leg with the arms stretched out in front, hands clasped together with index fingers in a steeple, pointing like an arrow.
2. The back leg stays straight and strong.
3. With a strong core, reach the arms overhead and finish in mountain. Switch supporting legs.

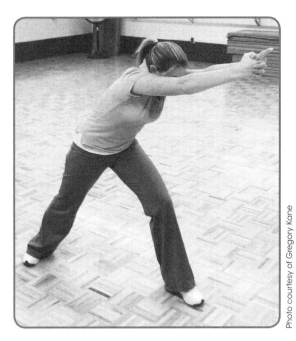

FIGURE 7.33   Arrow.

Photo courtesy of Gregory Kane

EAGLE

(can also be called noodle)

■ **Balancing Pose**

This pose is named after a bird in Indian folklore that never touches the earth but soars from beautiful tree bough to tree bough to rest. The eagle is a challenging pose, and it incorporates almost all the major joints of the body. It is important to keep the supporting leg bent so it is easier to wrap the other leg around the supporting leg (see figure 7.34).

Start

Begin in the mountain.

1. Squat down into chair, lift, and cross the left knee up and over the bent right knee.
2. Tell the students to pretend they are sitting in a chair with their legs tightly crossed.
3. Stretch the arms out to the side in airplane arms. Swing the left arm down and under the right arm, and wrap the forearms and wrists around each other.
4. Hold the elbows at shoulder height.
5. Keep the tailbone pointed down. Remind the students to use a focus point.
6. Unwrap the arms slowly. Stand up into mountain.
7. Repeat on the other side.

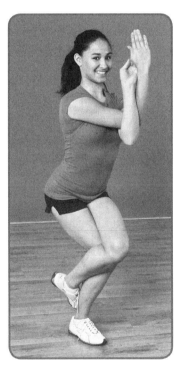

FIGURE 7.34   Eagle.

LIGHTHOUSE

■ **Balancing Pose, Grades 5+**

This pose resembles the movement of the light beam from a lighthouse as it slowly casts the light beam from side to side. This pose not only challenges balance but also our eye gaze moves and shifts, challenging us to remain calm and relaxed (see figure 7.35).

Start

Begin in mountain.

1. Standing on the right leg (supporting leg), arms straight out at the sides in airplane arms, lift the left knee to hip height (90 degrees), and hold it there.

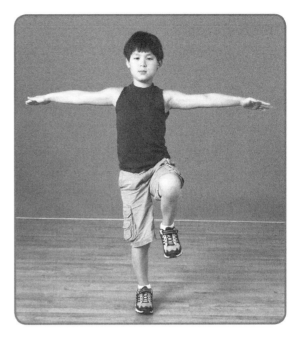

FIGURE 7.35 Lighthouse.

2. Slowly moving from the core, move the belly button to the right to spiral the upper body and airplane arms to the right, slowly shifting the eye gaze to look over the right shoulder.

3. Slowly spiral back to center, turn the upper body and airplane arms to the left, and look over the left shoulder.

4. Release to mountain and switch supporting legs.

STANDING BOW

(can also be called flamingo, stork, or dancer)

■ **Balancing Pose, Grades 3+**

Letting students hold onto a stationary object such as a chair or a wall may keep them from hopping around until they achieve balance in this fun balancing pose (see figure 7.36).

Start

Begin in mountain.

1. Standing on the right leg (supporting leg), bend the left leg at the knee, and reach back with the left hand to hold the left ankle or shin.

2. Reach up to the sky with the right arm, and hinge at the hip and bend forward.

3. Press the left foot into the left hand to create the shape of a bow. Hold and then release into mountain and switch feet.

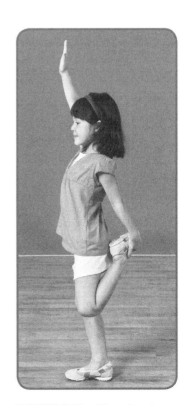

FIGURE 7.36 Standing bow.

TREE

- **Balancing Pose**

When you ask students what their favorite yoga pose is, they often give the same response: tree (see figure 7.37). We all love trees and enjoy emulating their strength and beauty.

Start

Begin in mountain.

1. Stand tall and strong, and place the weight on one leg (supporting leg). Tell the class to pretend the standing foot has grown roots into the earth below, and the top of the head is reaching to the sun.

2. Now bring the sole of the other foot to rest on the inner calf muscle or on the top of the supporting foot. Advanced students can place the sole of the foot on the inside of the upper thigh.

3. Tell students to keep their hands on the hips, hold their clasped hands at the chest, or slowly reach the arms overhead like limbs of a tree.

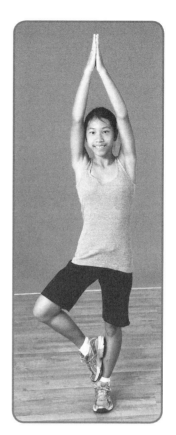

FIGURE 7.37 Tree.

4. Remind students to breathe and keep their eyes glued to a spot in front of them. Cue them by saying, "Remember your focus point!" and "Hold your tree pose strong and proud!"

5. Switch feet. Let the students use a chair or the wall if they need help balancing.

Infusion Idea

Say to the class, "What do trees give us? Leaves, fruit, nuts, wood for houses and furniture, and paper to write on. They give us oxygen so we can breathe!"

Discuss what the students can do to take care of trees (e.g., recycling newspapers and boxes, not being wasteful, not polluting the air—walking or riding bikes instead of driving).

WARRIOR III

(can also be called T pose or airplane)

- **Balancing Pose**

A lot of fun imagery can be used with warrior III, airplane, or T pose (see figure 7.38). Remind students to move slowly in and out of the pose and to keep their gaze on a fixed point (dhristi).

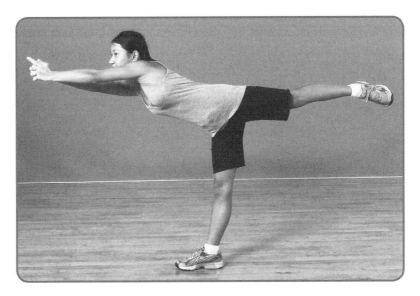

FIGURE 7.38   Warrior III.

Start

Begin in mountain.

1. Stand tall and strong on one leg (supporting leg). Take the arms out strong to the sides in airplane arms.

2. Balance on the supporting leg while lifting the other leg to the back. Hinge at the hips and tip forward.

3. Reach the arms forward to make a T, or keep the arms strong at the sides like the wings of an airplane.

4. Return to mountain.

5. Switch supporting legs.

> ▶ During the pose, you can cue students by saying, "You are an airplane soaring through the air. Can you come in for a landing by touching the ground in front and then gently lifting back up into airplane? Move your wings and soar!"

Infusion Idea

Ask the students where they would go in an airplane and what is special about that place (e.g., the language, things you can do there, animals that live there).

ACTIVE FLOOR POSES

Continue to challenge your students' health-related fitness by including poses that can still be active but are done on the floor. It is also important to watch the students' energy and to include some relaxing poses interspersed between the more-active poses so students can rest, recover, and feel balanced.

These poses are done on the floor but are still challenging and active. Keep reminding the students to be aware of their core muscles helping them in these floor poses.

BOAT

▪ **Active Floor Pose**

The boat challenges us to keep a strong core and not to slouch. Cue your students to keep the heart space lifted and the body in a strong V shape.

Start

Begin by sitting upright with the back straight and knees bent, feet flat on floor.

1. Lean back to balance between sitting bones and tailbone while lifting the knees and feet up parallel with the floor (see figure 7.39).

2. Arms are held at shoulder height, parallel with the floor or out to the side in airplane.

3. Keep the heart lifted so the body is a sharp V (don't slump), and balance.

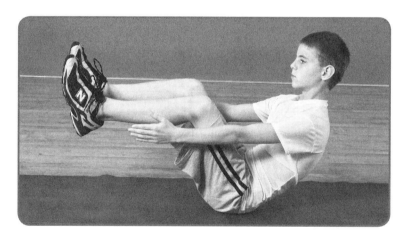

FIGURE 7.39 Boat.

Variation A: Full Boat

To advance, straighten the legs and arms so the whole body resembles a huge V.

Variation B: Row, Row, Row the Boat

Use the arms to row an imaginary boat.

Variation C: Jessica's Soup

Stay sitting up with the feet flat on the floor. Lean back, balancing between sitting bones and tailbone and keeping the heart space lifted. Tell the students to bring their hands together in front of the chest as if holding a big stirring spoon and make big circles as if stirring a huge bowl of soup.

BRIDGE

■ **Active Floor Pose**

The bridge is a pose that helps build strength in the core and legs. Ask the students to keep their eye gaze up at the ceiling and to pay attention and be mindful when lifting the hips up and resting on their shoulder blades (see figure 7.40).

Start

Begin while supine with the knees bent, hip-distance apart, and the feet under the hips, toes and knees pointed straight ahead.

1. Keep the arms alongside the body, with palms down.
2. Exhale and press the feet and lower back into the floor (cat tilt). Gently lift the hips off the ground, making a bridge with the back. Keep the breath flowing and strong.
3. Slowly lower the torso, beginning with the upper shoulders, shoulder blades, lower back, and gluteals.
4. Finish in nose to knees pose.

▶ Remind students to keep their eye gaze to the ceiling and not to turn the head. They can use their hands to support the small of their backs.

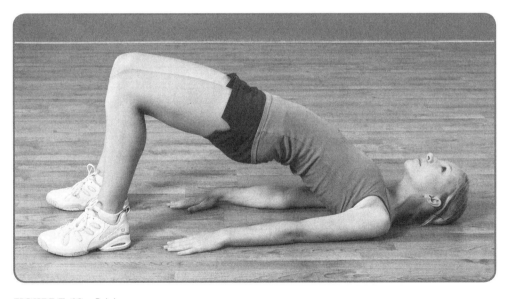

FIGURE 7.40 Bridge.

KNEELING BACK-BEND POSE

(can also be called camel)

- **Active Floor Pose**

This is a great chest opener and strengthens the back as well. Students may feel vulnerable with their heads back, so allow them to keep their eye gaze looking forward and their chins level with the ground if they need to.

Start

Begin from kneeling.

1. Place flat hands or fists to support the lower-back area (kidney area).
2. Push the hips forward, with gluteals strong.
3. Gently open the heart, and stretch into back bend.
4. Keep the hands at the back, or reach one arm up and back at a time, placing the fingertips on the ankles for balance (see figure 7.41).
5. Slowly release by reaching one arm at a time forward.

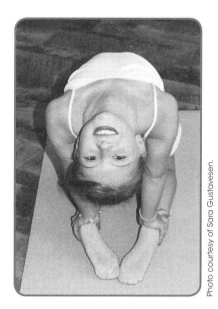

Photo courtesy of Sara Gustavesen.

FIGURE 7.41   Kneeling back bend.

LYING-DOWN BOW

- **Active Floor Pose**

Many students are flexible enough to do this pose easily (see figure 7.42), but it may be difficult for students who are heavy or have limited range of motion in the shoulders. Keep in mind that this pose can be done on one side only, lying facedown or standing up (see standing bow pose on page 137).

Start

Begin by lying prone (on the belly).

1. Bend both knees, reach back with both arms, and grab hold of the ankles from behind.
2. Engage the core muscles and lift the chest, head, and legs off the floor.
3. Press the ankles into the hands, creating a bow shape.
4. Slowly release.

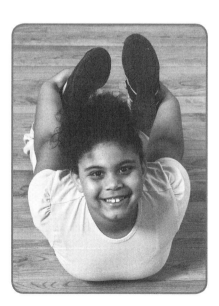

FIGURE 7.42   Lying-down bow.

Variation: Half Bow

Students can do the half bow—one side at a time lifts while the other side stays stable, glued to the ground.

PLANK

(can also be called pirate's plank or push-up)

⬛ **Active Floor Pose**

Set up the exercise by saying, "Think of a strong plank of wood you would use to walk from a boat to the dock. Make your whole body like this strong plank of wood" .

Start

From table pose, walk the knees back and lift up the legs so they are straight, the toes curled under while keeping the core engaged and the arms strong (see figure 7.43). Press the heart and crown of the head forward and the heels back.

Variation

The students can make a strong plank with their upper bodies but rest on the knees.

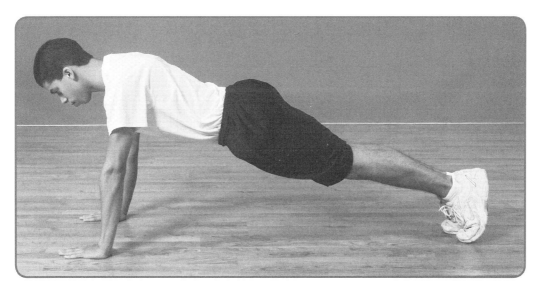

FIGURE 7.43 Plank.

REVERSE PLANK

(can also be called slide)

⬛ **Active Floor Pose**

The reverse plank is a nice counterpose to downward-facing dog or any core-intensive poses to allow the hips to move up and to strengthen the arms and legs.

Start

Begin sitting upright with the legs together and straight out in front.

1. Place the hands under the shoulders, keeping the fingers pointed toward the feet.

2. Keeping the legs together and firm, lift the hips up while planting the feet firmly into the ground (see figure 7.44).

3. Slowly release back to sitting.

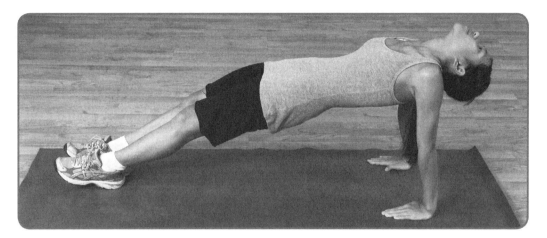

FIGURE 7.44   Reverse plank.

RIDE A BIKE

▪ **Active Floor Pose, Grades Pre-K-3**

This pose can help students engage and strengthen the abdominal muscles and also brings some movement into the active floor poses.

Start

Lying supine, bring the legs up over the hips. Lower the legs to 45 to 70 degrees, making sure the back is flat and supported by the floor. Begin to peddle the legs as if riding a bike (see figure 7.45). The arms can move in circles too.

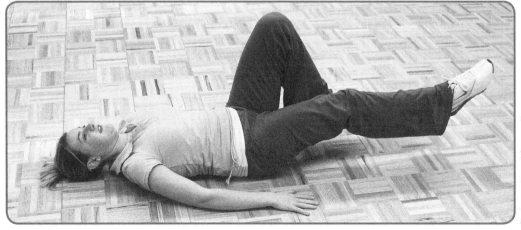

FIGURE 7.45   Ride a bike pose.

Photo courtesy of Gregory Kane.

SHARK

- **Active Floor Pose**

Here is another pose that engages the core and both the arms and legs. Do a resting pose such as windshield wipers (see page 153) to provide balance afterward.

Start

Lying prone (on the belly), engage the core muscles and lace the fingers behind the back, resembling a shark fin, to open the chest (see figure 7.46).

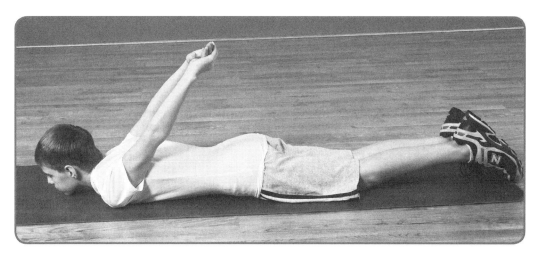

FIGURE 7.46   Shark.

SIDE PLANK

(can also be called rainbow)

- **Active Floor Pose, Grades 5+**

This is a wonderful pose to challenge core strength and to keep the whole core and body strong and engaged (see figure 7.47).

Start

Start from push-up.

1. Shift the weight onto the right hand, and roll onto the side of the right foot.
2. Stretch the left arm up to the sky.
3. The left foot can rest on top of the right, or the feet can be staggered.
4. Slowly release back to front plank or table, and do the other side.

Variation

Instead of keeping the right leg straight, bend the right knee for balance, and balance on the bent knee for support.

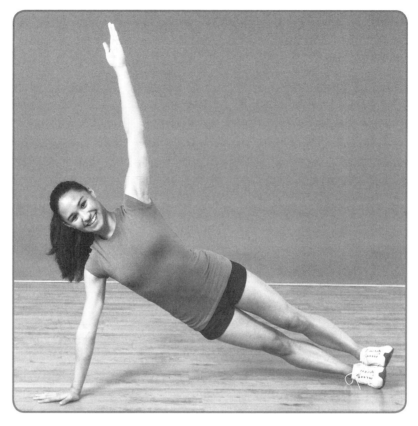

FIGURE 7.47 Side plank.

SUPERHERO

▪ **Active Floor Pose**

This pose allows all the muscles to work at once. Do a resting pose afterward, and give students time to practice "letting go of the pose," meaning it may take a few extra relaxing breaths for them to completely let go after engaging the legs, the arms, and so on.

Start

Begin by lying supine (face up).

1. Extend and lengthen both arms and legs, engage the core of body, and lift the arms and legs 2-3 inches (5-8 centimeters) from the floor. Hold.

2. Gently lower both arms and legs (see figure 7.48). Roll over and bend the knees to slowly sweep the legs back and forth (like a windshield wiper) to release the body.

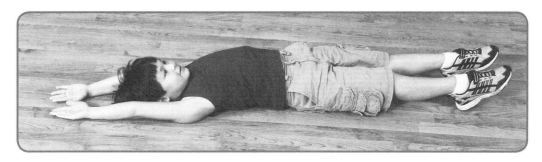

FIGURE 7.48 Superhero.

Variation A

Modify by doing only legs or only arms.

Variation B: Swimming

Lying prone (on the belly), lift the arms and legs 2-3 inches (5-8 centimeters) from the ground. Gently imitate swimming by alternating one leg and arm higher than the other in a fluttering motion.

Variation C: Grasshopper

Lying prone, lift both legs while strongly reaching the arms back toward the toes 2-3 inches (5-8 centimeters) off the floor (see figure 7.49).

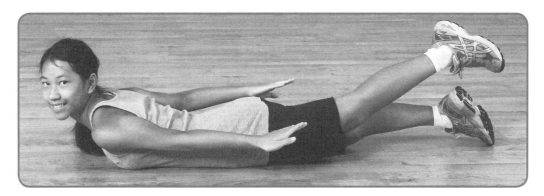

FIGURE 7.49 Grasshopper.

Variation D: Crocodile

Lying prone, reach the arms in front together, opening and closing like a crocodile's jaw, while keeping the legs firmly together on the floor, swishing them side to side like a crocodile's tail.

Infusion Idea

Ask the students, "Who are some heroes who help us every day? How can we be everyday heroes to our families, school, friends, and community?"

COOL-DOWN POSES

After you have worked hard in your floor poses, start the cool-down phase of your yoga practice. However, the cool-down poses are not reserved for just the cool-down but can be used as counterposes after challenging poses. Teaching students to be able to put forth a strong effort and equally pay attention to relaxing and allowing the body to rest gives them an important skill they can use away from the yoga mat as well. By paying close attention to the students' energy level, especially when the challenging poses can be very stimulating, you give the students the chance to let go and move on from the challenge and stay present in the next pose or activity. These quieting poses allow for this to happen.

Please note that the following cool-down poses can also be offered as ways to slowly quiet down after an active session, can be interspersed between active poses, can be used as modifications when students need a less-active pose, and can be used for a class devoted to relaxation poses when your students need a break.

BUTTERFLY

▪ **Cool-Down Pose**

This is a great hip flexor stretch.

Start

Begin seated, with the back straight and strong.

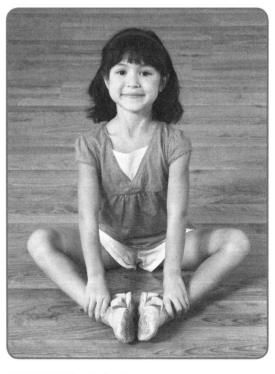

1. Bend the knees and open them out to the sides like butterfly wings. Let the legs gently flap like a butterfly on the breeze.
2. Hold onto the feet, and bring the bottoms of the feet together. Turn the soles of the feet to face the ceiling (see figure 7.50).
3. Fold forward from the hips and hold.

Variation A: Half Butterfly

One leg remains straight while the other knee drops into butterfly.

Variation B: Reclined Butterfly

FIGURE 7.50 Butterfly pose.

Perform the pose on the back, with the knees dropped out to the sides. Blankets or yoga blocks can be placed under the knees for support.

Infusion Idea

Ask the students what butterflies do to help our gardens and farmers.

FETAL

(can also be called reflection pose)

■ **Cool-Down Pose**

The fetal pose is an important pose to use frequently as it allows the back to release by drawing the knees in.

Start

Lying on the back, gently roll onto the side of the body, bringing the knees toward the chest and allowing the upper arms to rest comfortably by either hugging the knees or resting the head on folded hands, making a pillow (see figure 7.51).

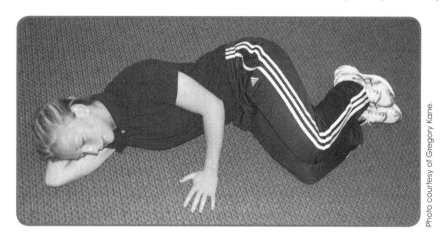

Photo courtesy of Gregory Kane.

FIGURE 7.51 Fetal.

HAPPY BABY

■ **Cool-Down Pose**

Remind your students that when they were babies, they could all do the happy baby pose—they could even put their feet in their mouths!

Start

Begin by lying supine (on the back).

1. Lift both knees up and into the chest, and open the knees out to the sides.

2. Reach both arms through the legs, grab hold of the toes or shins, and allow the body to relax (see figure 7.52).

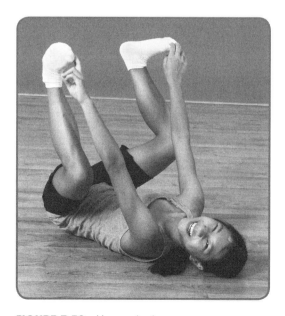

FIGURE 7.52 Happy baby.

Infusion Idea

Say to the class, "You used to be able to do this easily. You could even put your toes in your mouth! What happened? We need to stay flexible by doing yoga!"

SEATED STRAIGHT-LEG FORWARD FOLD

▪ **Cool-Down Pose**

It is very soothing for the body to be put into a forward fold pose.

Start

Sit up straight with the legs in front, feet flexed (toes pointed to the sky); the legs and feet are engaged and active.

1. Reach up to the sky with both arms, and fold at the hips, keeping the back strong (not collapsing). Do not slouch, making sure the thoracic and lumbar spines are strong but letting the cervical spine (the neck area) release by letting the chin drop to the chest (see figure 7.53).

2. Hold onto the shins or ankles, and allow the hamstrings to lengthen.

Variation

Hold both ends of a towel wrapped around the bottom of the feet if it is too difficult to reach toward the legs.

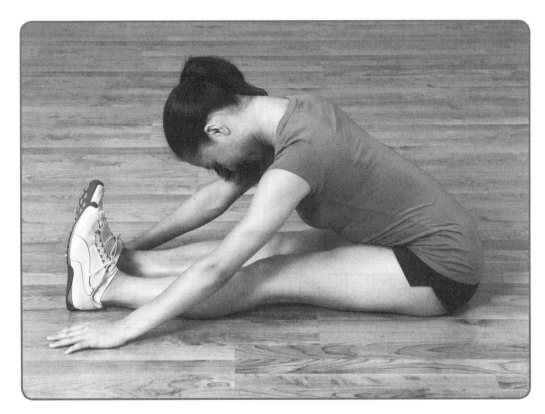

FIGURE 7.53 Seated straight-leg forward fold.

SEATED TWIST

▪ **Cool-Down Pose**

This pose brings in the element of spiraling the spine. Remind the students to maintain strong posture in this pose with an engaged core and to mindfully start the spiral, or twist, from the tailbone and slowly work upward through the spine, never forcing or stressing the back.

Start

Begin seated, with the legs straight out in front.

1. Keeping one leg glued to the floor and sitting tall, bend the other knee and cross that leg over the straight leg, drawing it close to the chest while keeping the foot on the floor, and hug the bent knee with the opposite hand.

2. Slowly turn the belly button toward the bent knee, and slowly spiral (turn) the shoulder and chest toward the bent knee while still hugging the knee. Reach back with the other arm (see figure 7.54).

3. Come back to center. Switch legs.

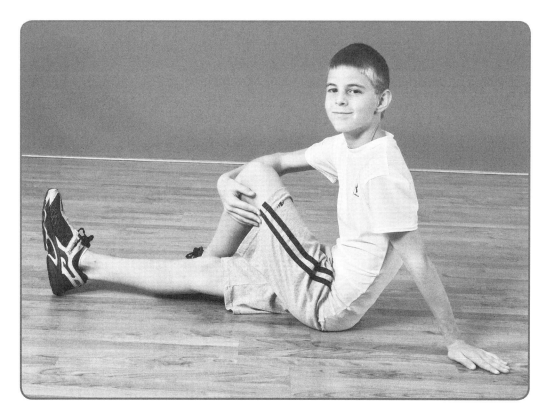

FIGURE 7.54 Seated twist.

TURTLE

▧ **Cool-Down Pose**

This pose reminds us of an important lesson in life: A turtle does not go fast but moves steadily toward his goal. Encourage students not to strive to make their turtle stance as wide as possible, but to keep it only 2-3 feet (.6 to .9 meter) wide.

Start

Sit up tall. Separate the feet about as wide as the yoga mat, 2 to 3 feet (.6 to .9 meter) apart.

1. Reach the arms overhead and hinge at the hips. Reach forward and hold onto the toes, shins, or ankles (see figure 7.55). Keep the knees soft—as bent as needed.

2. Bend a little more forward, and feel the stretch. Tell the students to let their necks be long, like a turtle's head coming out of its shell.

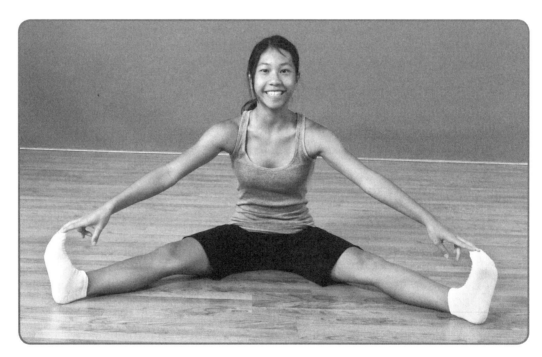

FIGURE 7.55   Turtle.

Infusion Idea

Say to the class, "Think about a goal you might have, such as getting a good grade in math. What do you need to do to reach your goals? Practice! That is what we do in yoga—we practice a little bit each time, and we slowly, like the turtle, reach our goal of being healthy and happy."

WINDSHIELD WIPERS

▧ Cool-Down Pose

This pose is a great lower-back release, but caution the students to move their legs slowly side to side, as if there is a light mist and not a heavy downpour.

Start

This pose can be done either while lying on the belly or sitting up on the floor.

1. While lying on the belly, bend at the knees; the feet stay up in the air. Let the legs slowly swish side to side to release the back (see figure 7.56).

2. While seated, the arms are behind to offer support, with the knees bent and as wide apart as the mat. Slowly drop the knees to one side. Change direction, allowing the knees to drop to the other side.

Variation

Do the pose while lying on the back.

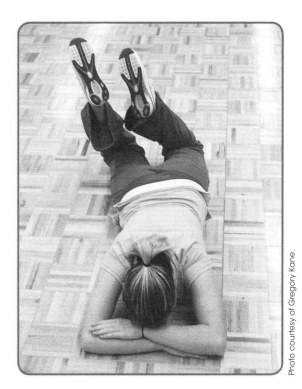

Photo courtesy of Gregory Kane.

FIGURE 7.56 Windshield wipers.

SUMMARY

How many poses you use in a class will depend on the age and developmental level of the students, the yoga space you have available, and how much time you have for your class. When first introducing yoga to a group of students, perhaps use four to six basic poses with younger students and maybe six to eight basic poses with older students that they all will learn as a core; add one or two new poses each class. Try to experiment as much as possible while giving yourself full permission to explore different ways to creatively vary the poses. Ask students to make up their own poses—individually, with partners, or in small groups. As stated previously, there are countless poses and variations, with equally countless names. Students may also have their own favorites they have tried or seen. If you prefer not to do a pose in class, feel free to say, "Thank you for the suggestion, but we will not be doing that pose in class."

The next chapter provides ideas for infusing themes and academic topics into yoga class, indoor recess, or anywhere. This chapter and the next do not provide an exhaustive list of every game or activity to use during yoga but are intended to act as a catalyst for instructors to come up with their own unique and wonderful ideas for teaching yoga.

chapter

8

Infusing Themes Into Yoga Classes

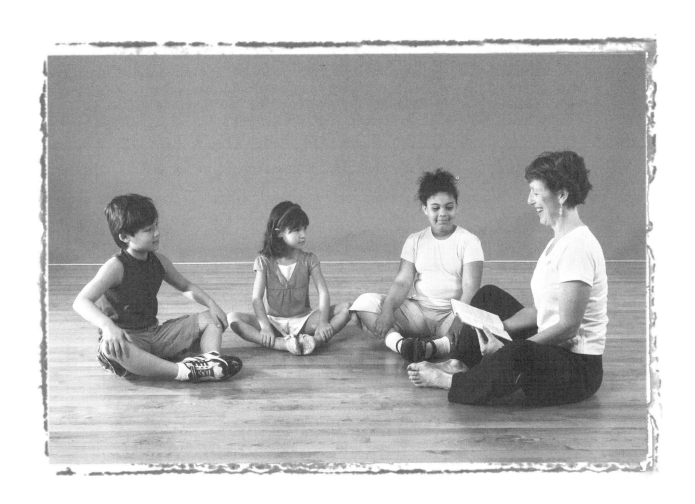

Yoga is a lifelong practice of healthy and balanced living. The teachings of yoga are universal and will help students enjoy a holistic activity that integrates the body, the spirit, and the mind. Yoga games offered here are examples of traditional games that can be adapted to include yoga poses and allow all students to be included. This chapter provides ideas of thematic topics that can inspire the connections to healthy and balanced living and yoga. These themes cover important areas of the growth and development of your students, including self-image, healthy habits, getting along and working with others, creative problem solving, and making the world a better place. The last section includes ways to infuse yoga into academic subjects such as art, literacy, and science.

This chapter provides general ideas for all ages. Some adaptations and recommendations are included for younger students (generally preschool through elementary) and older students (generally middle or junior high through the teenage years). Keep in mind that play is essential for all ages. For that reason, it is important that all students adopt an attitude of having fun instead of focusing on how they look or whether they are doing things right. The goal should be looking inward and letting go of individual constraints and self-imposed limitations.

There are countless ways to infuse and integrate themes and academic areas into yoga classes. Activities can be as simple as making alphabet shapes or numbers with the body to discussing the angles of a triangle in math while doing the triangle pose. Examples of ways to enhance student learning and yoga with younger students are making crafts, using picture books and music, or using puppets. With older students, activities could include journal writing, group discussion, making posters or murals, mentoring with younger students, service projects, and creating yoga board games. This final chapter asks you, the instructor, to adopt the yoga philosophy of being open by trying some of the activities presented, adapting them to your students' needs, or adapting your own activities. Your students will thank you for it!

YOGA GAMES

Many traditional games for younger students can be adapted to include yoga. These games should be played with the goal of cooperation and inclusion, not competition and eliminating students. Just adapt the rules to allow a student to be the leader, and then pass the leadership onto another student. Let the students know that everyone gets a turn in all the games they play together. Older elementary students (grades 3 to 5) tend to be very dependent on rules, and so focusing away from rules and more on everyone participating is a critical concept to reinforce.

The game examples here are just the tip of the iceberg of creative ways to infuse healthy living principles; academic lessons; and a variety of movement experiences, imagination, and, most important, fun into yoga classes. To find more creative physical education games, visit the physical education Web sites in the resource section.

CHIME TIME

▪ **Yoga Game for Younger Students**

The students sit in a circle in a cross-legged seated pose, with the eyes closed. One student walks quietly around the circle and gently rings a small bell behind one of the students. They change places, and now the new student walks quietly with the bell. This game helps students sit quietly but stay alert.

CRAZY FROGS

▪ **Yoga Game for Younger Students**

Students begin by jumping like frogs around the yoga space. When you give a signal or stop the music, each student finds a partner, and they squat back to back with their hands out in front for balance. When you call out, "Crazy frogs," the students lift up their gluteals, fold forward in wide-angle forward fold pose, and look at their partners between their legs with a big froggy smile. Give another signal or start the music again, telling the frogs to jump away until it's time to find a new partner.

DOGS IN A ROW

▪ **Yoga Game for Younger Students**

1. Everyone in the group does downward-facing dog in a row, making a tunnel that one student crawls through without touching anyone (see figure 8.1). You may need to break the class into groups so that the one student can get through the down dog tunnel before it collapses.

2. The whole group does child pose or another relaxing pose. Then it is the next student's turn to crawl.

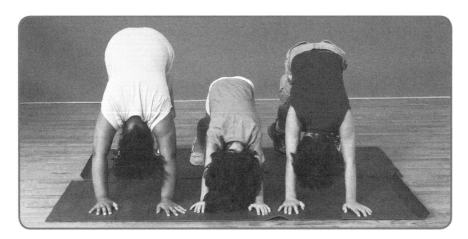

FIGURE 8.1 Dogs in a row.

DRIVING THE CAR

▪ **Yoga Game for Younger Students**

Tell the students to use their arms as steering wheels, with feet on the brakes, while in boat pose. The students can move around the room in their car, bus, or tractor.

ELEPHANT, ELEPHANT—LEADER OF THE JUNGLE

▪ **Yoga Game for Younger Students**

One student is the lead elephant in the middle of the circle. All the students come into elephant pose (holding onto their wrists and swinging their arms side to side like an elephant's trunk) while walking in the circle. The lead elephant states a pose, and all the other elephants freeze into that pose. Then it is someone else's turn to be the lead elephant.

ROLLER COASTER

▪ **Yoga Game for Younger Students**

The students come into turtle pose, one lined up behind the other in a row, and can hold onto the shoulders of the student in front of them (see figure 8.2). The roller coaster can move by leaning back, moving forward, and moving right or left.

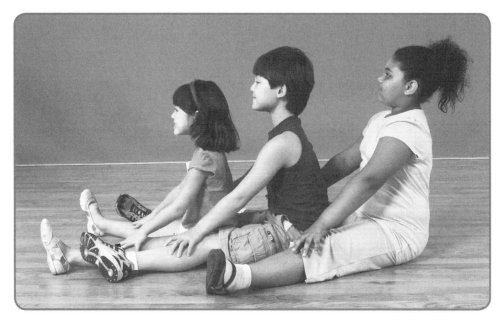

FIGURE 8.2 Roller coaster.

OODLES OF NOODLES

▪ **Yoga Game**

Noodles are pieces of foam used to help swimmers float in the water. They cost very little and are virtually indestructible. They can also be used as colorful markers to delineate a space. These activities are a fun way for students to use various locomotor skills. In this activity, noodles are spread around the activity space.

Part One

Each time a student approaches a noodle she may jump, hop, leap, or do a fancy jump over it or place her hands on the floor over the noodle and transfer her weight back and forth over it, doing a cartwheel.

Part Two

Add music to the activity. When you stop the music, students find a noodle and incorporate it into a yoga pose, such as tipping star or warrior II (see figure 8.3); perform a yoga pose over the noodle, such as bridge or downward-facing dog (see figure 8.4); or freeze, making a funny statue using the noodle.

Part Three

1. Students pick up a noodle and go to their yoga mats to follow along with a story. Set up the exercise by saying, "Today we are going to travel with our noodles all over the world!"

2. Cue students by saying, "We are off to the jungle, and we will see

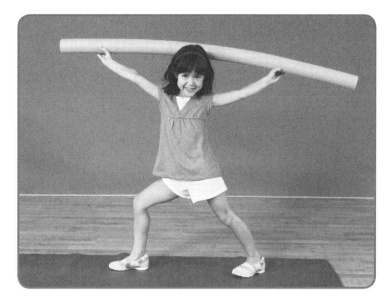

FIGURE 8.3 Using a noodle in the warrior II pose.

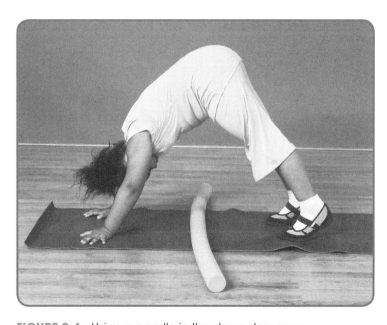

FIGURE 8.4 Using a noodle in the down dog pose.

an elephant [students make a trunk with their noodles]. There is a snake [students hold onto one end of the noodle while moving it in a snakelike motion]. Let's travel back in time and make a dinosaur with a big tail [students make dinosaur tails with their noodles]. Let's make a unicorn [students place the noodles on the forehead]."

Variations

Other ways to use the noodle include marching in a parade where the noodle is a baton; pretending to be circus performers by balancing the noodle on different parts of the body (see figure 8.5); or riding a horse with the noodle between the legs.

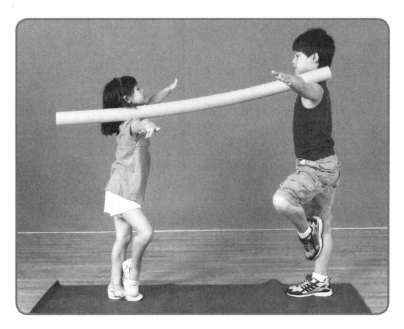

FIGURE 8.5 Balancing a noodle in the circus.

RED LIGHT, GREEN LIGHT

▨ **Yoga Game**

1. One student is the light keeper and stands at the front of the yoga space, facing away from the class. The other students line up at the other end of the yoga space.

2. The light keeper starts the game by stating, "Green light." The other students slowly start to move toward the light keeper. The movement can be predetermined such as tiptoeing, skipping, crawling, hopping, or spinning.

3. The light keeper turns to face the group and at the same time states, "Red light."

4. All of the group freeze into any yoga pose or a predetermined yoga pose such as tree.

5. Any students who do not freeze start over again at the start line.

6. If someone from the group reaches the light keeper and taps him, she becomes the light keeper, and the light keeper joins the group at the start line to start a new round.

Younger Students

There may need to be a predetermined amount of time the light keeper is in charge, as it may be difficult for the students to freeze without moving.

ROBOT DOING YOGA

■ **Yoga Game**

Students can mimic robotlike moves while doing various yoga poses. Or try another theme, such as Ninja Turtles, Harry Potter, or rock stars doing yoga.

TWELVE DAYS OF YOGA

■ **Yoga Game**

Everyone sings to the tune of "The Twelve Days of Christmas."
 On the first day of yoga, my teacher gave to me

12 tipping stars,

11 quarter moons,

10 claps and stamps (hopping in place and clapping hands),

9 "I-don't-knows" (shoulder shrugs),

8 warrior IIs (switching side to side from warrior II right to warrior II left),

7 jumping jacks,

6 standing twisters (standing twists side to side),

5 dragon snorts (blowing air out nose with lips sealed),

4 sitting chairs (sitting down into chair pose and back up to standing),

3 forward dives (arms in airplane, folding forward to hip height, and standing tall again),

2 lion roars,

and an eagle sitting in a tree (eagle).

YOGI SAYS

■ **Yoga Game**

One student is the yogi (the name for a student of yoga), and the rest of the students listen carefully to the pose "Yogi says" to do (similar to the game Simon says).

YOGA STATIONS

Stations are a great way for students to do a variety of activities as they move from station to station after a specific period of time or a certain number of repetitions of a movement or pose. You can set up stations in a circle or in different corners of the room. A cone or a noodle can mark each station, where a card with a picture or stick figure and simple directions of the movement or pose can be displayed. Mix yoga poses in with the movements so the students stay active. Yoga blocks or blankets can be available at the stations to help students with the poses. Divide the students into teams for each of the stations you have. Make sure there is enough space and equipment at each station. You can set a timer for a certain amount of time at each session to signal the students to proceed to the next station.

YOGA JIVE FIVE

▪ **Yoga Stations**

Everything in this station circuit example is based on the number five (see figure 8.6).

- Station one: Hold tree pose on each leg for five breaths.
- Station two: Do 5 × 5 (25) jumping jacks.
- Station three: Do teeter-totter five times (back and forth between warrior II and extended side angle or reverse warrior).
- Station four: Swing the hula hoop five times to the left and five times to the right.
- Station five: Sit in chair pose for five breaths.

When the students finish all the stations, they can be repeated.

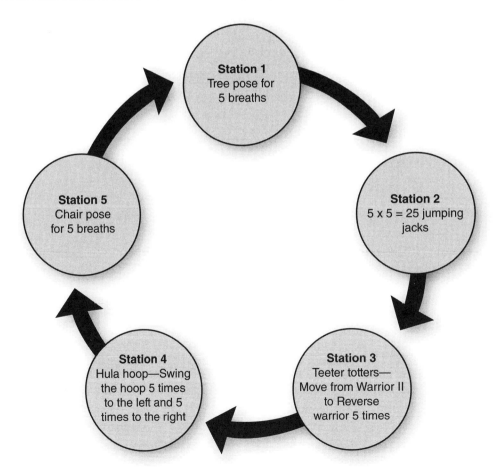

FIGURE 8.6 Yoga Jive Five.

SELF-IMAGE AND YOGA

Yoga is an experiential activity for individual growth and development. When yoga is presented in a fun, inclusive, and open manner, the students' self-image will be affected in positive ways. This in turn influences the other important areas of your students' growth and development, such as getting along with others and having the confidence to do well in academic areas.

MY FAVORITE YOGA POSE

▪ Self-Image Activity

Ask students to draw pictures of themselves doing their favorite poses. Students can include words or phrases that convey how doing the pose makes them feel, such as *strong, happy, silly, content, at peace* (see figure 8.7).

Older Students

Older students can do self-portraits that show how they feel practicing yoga.

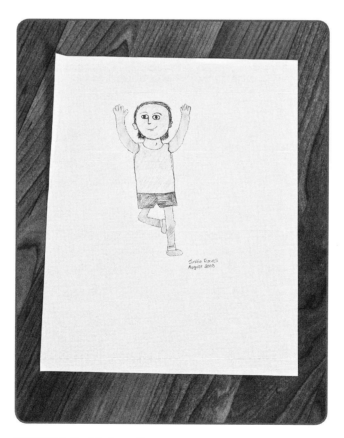

FIGURE 8.7 My favorite yoga pose.

GORILLA

■ **Self-Image Activity**

This activity can be done while lying down, standing, or sitting. Gorilla allows the students to open up their throats and lungs and release some tension in the chest and neck area. For some students, it is great to be able to hear their voices when they might not be encouraged or feel reluctant to do so in class. If you watch young children at play, you'll notice that they scream or squeal as a means of just releasing tension and showing delight and energy in what they are doing.

Younger Students

Instruct younger students to gently tap on their chests as they use their bellies to make a sustained roar that is long but not loud. Lion's roar is another good release exercise (see page 90).

Older Students

Gorilla can also be called Shake It Off. Students gently tap, stretch, and shake the arms, legs, and head while making audible sighing noises and exhaling to release some pent-up tension.

"I FEEL GOOD ABOUT"

■ **Self-Image Activity**

At the end of class, students sit in a circle ready to contribute to the closing circle's theme or question. Sitting in this closing circle, students state one thing they like about themselves. Or students can decorate a poster or T-shirt with words that describe themselves.

Younger Students

1. Sitting in a closing circle, students discuss how we are all different, including the importance of diversity in nature. What would it be like if all flowers were the same colors, if all food were the same, or if all the animals were the same?

2. Ask the students to identify some reasons for diversity (e.g., shapes of leaves, colors for protection).

Older Students

Students discuss in a closing circle or reflect in a journal entry their strengths and how being different and respecting and learning more about how others differ are important.

SELF-AFFIRMATION

▪ **Self-Image Activity**

Affirmations are positive statements that are repeated over and over. Students think of their own statements or use examples that you provide. The statement should be written in an affirming, positive form and in the present tense. This can be a difficult task because so much of a student's self-talk is modeled on negativity such as "I can't," "I have to," or "I am not able." You may need to guide the students in tweaking their statements. For example, a student might write "I will not overeat or pig out." To shift the focus of this statement to an affirmation statement, it could be written as "I am making healthy eating choices that I enjoy."

Younger Students

Post examples of affirmations around the room so students can read them often and start to use the positive language of affirmative statements. The quintessential story of "the little engine that could" is a user-friendly example of affirmations.

Older Students

Sometimes older students find using affirmations awkward at first—these students are not accustomed to using positive statements. Providing examples that use words that are authentic to the students can help inspire them. Students can write out their affirmations on index cards or make screen savers for their computers to remind them of their affirmation statements.

SELF-AFFIRMATION MEDITATION

▪ **Self-Image Activity**

This meditation can be done seated or during relaxation.

1. On the inhale, tell the students to say to themselves, "I am."

2. On the exhale, tell the students to complete the statement with something positive: happy, strong, confident, motivated, prepared, a good friend, getting stronger every day, working toward my goals.

The exercises in this section are just a few ways to focus on improving the self-esteem of your students. Yoga intuitively brings out confidence and positive feelings and is a natural tool to help build self-esteem. Self-esteem is a necessary part of living a healthy lifestyle—when you care about yourself in positive ways, you will seek ways to feel better in positive ways as well.

HEALTHY LIFESTYLE AND YOGA

You can use yoga to encourage students to engage in everyday practices that make them healthy inside and out. What is amazing about practicing positive ways to live a healthy and balanced life is that everything interconnects and has synergy. For example, if you eat well you feel better and have more energy for being active, which then helps you sleep better. By helping students incorporate small but significant steps on the path to healthy and balanced living, you will help them develop a positive relationship with themselves that will stay with them for a lifetime.

BRAINSTORMING WAYS WE CAN BE HEALTHIER EVERY DAY

▪ **Healthy Lifestyle Exercise**

Brainstorming is a method that allows the students to spontaneously come up with ideas to solve a problem. There are no wrong ideas, and students can help each other fine-tune their ideas to solve the problem better.

Following are some ideas for brainstorming ways to be healthier every day:

- Use positive building statements, not put-downs.
- Ask for help.
- Perform 60 minutes of physical activity every day.
- Take a stretch break.
- Take a walk.
- Do your own work, and do your best.
- Get enough sleep.
- Volunteer!
- Limit your "electronic time" to 2 hours or less each day.
- Jump rope.
- Eat fruit for a snack.
- Recycle.
- Help out at home.
- Drink enough water.
- Share.
- Clean up after yourself.
- Take five full, deep breaths when your buttons get pushed.
- Read a book.
- Do your chores without being told.
- Look out for your friends.

- Say please.
- Show up with a positive attitude.
- Ask before you take something.
- Smile and make a new friend.
- Listen to your classmates.
- Say thank you.
- Get some quiet time.
- Help your friends.
- Brush and floss.
- Be kind in your words.
- Respect others' space, time, and energy.
- Eat five servings of vegetables each day.
- Spend time with a trusted adult.

GRATITUDE MEDITATION

■ **Healthy Lifestyle Meditation**

This meditation is a wonderful way to cultivate looking for gratitude in students' lives. Gratitude themes can include being grateful for teachers, our school, learning, friends, pets, our community, and activities that make us healthy and happy.

HEALTHY AND HAPPY HEARTS

■ **Healthy Lifestyle Exercise**

"You can have a healthy heart; it's as easy as 1, 2, 3! Eat healthy food, move your body, and live tobacco-free." This is the American Heart Association's motto for having a healthy heart.

1. Ask the students to make up poses that represent healthy food choices.
2. Students then do movements mimicking their favorite physical activity.
3. As the students do standing balloon breath, talk about how great it is to breathe easily, and the way to do that is to "live tobacco-free." The American Heart Association has other teaching materials for all ages on their Web site.
4. Ask the students to sit quietly and count their pulses, then take some relaxing breaths or do a relaxation exercise and recount the pulse. Students can see that by doing these activities, they can self-regulate their hearts and make them healthy and happy.

HEART-CENTERED MEDITATION

▫ **Healthy Lifestyle Meditation**

This is an appropriate activity for the close of yoga class or anytime the students need a break. Ask the students to sit quietly for a few moments and breathe as if breathing in and out of the heart space. Pick an intention for the meditation. Some intentions for heart-centered meditation might be gratitude, empathy, caring, friends, sharing, or listening. Ask the students to think of the meaning of this word in their life or picture things they are grateful for or come up with words that describe a good friend. Students can draw or write about their heart-centered meditation as well. If your students are struggling with a concept in class such as bullying or not sharing, ask them to focus on positive ways to deal with the issue in a nonthreatening and heart-centered way.

Older Students

Connecting this meditation with journal writing or art is a great way for older students to reflect on the importance of coming out of their heads and into a more heart-centered approach to the issues of their lives. See the resource section about HeartMath from the Institute of HeartMath, which is an organization advocating the importance of heart-centered activities for all ages.

SANDWICHES

▫ **Healthy Lifestyle Exercise**

The students are either standing or seated and come into forward fold, making "sandwiches." Discuss their favorite sandwiches and ways to make the sandwiches healthier (e.g., adding vegetables).

TAKE HEART

▫ **Healthy Lifestyle Exercise**

This activity includes discussion about the heart:

- What does the heart do?
- Where is it? How big is it?
- What can we do to make it stronger?
- What do we do that makes it weaker?

After the discussion, you will give several examples, and the students will decide whether each example makes the heart stronger or weaker. If the example makes the heart stronger, the students do the warrior pose; if the example makes the heart weaker, they will melt into the floor in a heap.

Here are some examples:

- Ride a bike? Sitting all day in front of the computer?
- Doing something nice for someone? Using a put-down statement?
- Eating fresh vegetables? Driving in a car when you could walk?
- Eating fast food all the time? Drinking soda pop instead of water?

INTERPERSONAL RELATIONSHIPS AND YOGA

One of the most important lessons in yoga is nonharming, known in Sanskrit as Ahimsa. It is hard for students to learn to take care of each other when it may not be modeled in the media, their community, or their home situations. There is never enough time spent on reinforcing taking care of each other and resolving conflicts in positive ways. The poses and activities offered here are experiential activities to help students work on empathy, active listening, cooperation, patience, and sharing with their peers.

Helping students find ways to enjoy working and learning cooperatively with each other is a gift that will carry over to many other aspects of their lives throughout the life span.

DANCING TURTLES

■ **Interpersonal Relationships and Yoga**

Two students face each other with feet apart and touching, holding onto each other's hands. One partner gently folds forward into turtle as the other partner gently leans back. Students can reach to the sides and up and down (see figure 8.8).

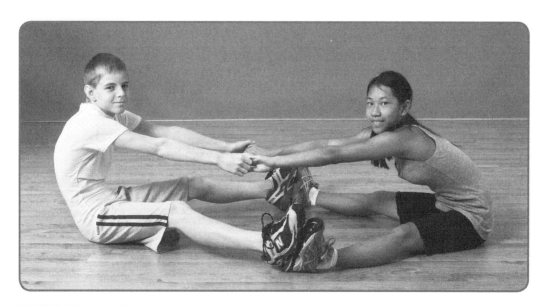

FIGURE 8.8 Dancing turtles.

IMAGINATION YOGA

▨ **Interpersonal Relationships and Yoga**

Students work in partners or small groups to create new poses.

PEACEKEEPER CORNER

▨ **Interpersonal Relationships and Yoga**

Have a designated place, such as a worktable, that students can go to when they are angry. This table can have materials to allow students to proactively deal with their strong emotions such as paper, pens, colors, a puzzle, stress balls, or music. When they are finished, they need to be assured that they can rejoin the class and are welcomed back. It is important to reinforce their decision to take themselves out of a stressful situation, regroup, and then join the class again.

PEACEKEEPER SPELLING BEE

▨ **Interpersonal Relationships and Yoga**

The students define and use in context the vocabulary of peacekeeping.
   Spelling bee words for younger students: apologize, communicate, compromise, confidential, conflict resolution, fighting fair, bully, victim, building statements, put-down statements, courage, abuse, friends
   Spelling bee words for older students: bystanders, assertiveness, negotiation, mediation, passiveness, aggression, emotional coercion, cultural norms, discriminate, cliques, exclusion, inclusion, resiliency

WARRIOR KNOW-HOW

▨ **Interpersonal Relationships and Yoga**

The warrior poses are strong metaphors for students being peacekeepers. Hold a discussion that focuses on ways students can be advocates for important issues in their lives for healthy and balanced living. Some healthy lifestyle advocacy topics include keeping physical education classes fun; new equipment for their gym; the importance of recess; having the cafeteria offer healthy food choices; time for quiet reading at school; no tolerance for bullying, cliques, or cyberbullies; setting up recycling stations; legislation for no smoking in cars with children; setting up peer mediation at their school; students mentoring younger grades; and making a designated yoga space at their school.

Older Students

Older students can select class projects such as blogs, Web sites, posters, murals, or debates; write letters to officials or the school board; or make PSAs (public service announcements), newsletters, or brochures. Service learning projects are ways the older students can serve their community. Mentoring younger students, going into the classrooms of younger students and role-playing ways to resolve conflicts, and doing other forms of community service are valuable experiential learning experiences.

FIGHTING FAIR

■ Getting Along With Others

In yoga we practice the principle of Ahimsa, which means nonharming. We do not harm ourselves or others. Have a discussion with the class:

- What are some ways we can be fair with people we may not agree with? Listen, find out the problem, care about each other's feelings, be responsible for what we say and do, realize we do not have to be right or to win, use building statements.

- Why do we use rules? So that everyone knows how to act in ways that help each other.

- What are some ways of not fighting fair? These are called fouls or bad habits: blaming, making excuses, booing, not listening, teasing, threatening in words or actions, using put-down statements, or using disrespectful body language.

- Are there some fouls you use often?

- Think about something that bugs you—how could you better handle this situation using the rules for fighting fair?

MEDIATION

■ Getting Along With Others

A mediator is a person who doesn't take sides but is an impartial listener and advocate who helps the two parties reach an agreement. It is confidential and on a volunteer basis for all parties involved, including the mediator. There is no blame assigned or winner determined; rather, mediation is a means of solving the problem. The mediator asks each of the two parties to answer the following questions (each party takes a turn answering the questions, while the other party listens without interrupting):

1. What is the problem?
2. What are you feeling?

The mediator then asks each party to brainstorm ways the problem can be resolved. During this process, it should be remembered that the parties are only brainstorming ideas and there are no wrong or stupid suggestions. The mediator only asks for ideas and does not offer his or her own solutions to the problem.

After all the ideas have been offered by the two parties, the mediator asks each party to focus on finding a solution that both parties state they will commit to. An agreement can be verbal or written down and witnessed by the mediator.

Partner Poses

Partner poses are a great way for older students to work together and communicate. Parents can do poses with their children for a nice bonding activity. Instruct students on proper ways to touch and ask for help from a partner. There are hundreds of different ways to do partner poses, and the following examples will hopefully spark some creative juices for other potential poses.

ASSISTED COBRA STRETCH-OUT

▨ **Partner Pose**

One student lies on the floor in cobra, with the arms alongside the body. The partner straddles the cobra, facing the same way, and gently assists by lifting and holding the cobra's shoulders or wrists and gently stretching them back (see figure 8.9).

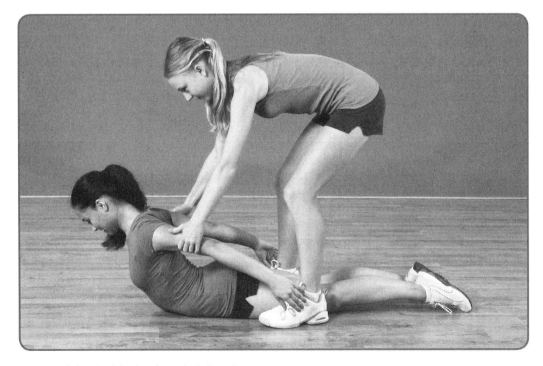

FIGURE 8.9 Assisted cobra stretch-out.

BACK TO BACK

■ **Partner Pose**

Start

Standing back to back, students do triangle, warrior II, tree, or standing wide-angle forward fold with their backs each supporting the other, or they can each move in the opposite direction and still support each other.

For example, in standing wide-angle forward fold pose, students stand back to back. Students fold forward into standing wide-angle forward fold and reach through their legs and hold onto each other's wrists.

BACK-TO-BACK SEATED POSES

■ **Partner Pose**

Start

Students sit cross-legged with their backs against each other as they feel each other's breath in the back of their bodies. From here they can gently twist the same way and hold this seated twist pose, then switch to gently twist the other way. Sitting back to back again, students can take turns making different noises, and the partner feels the resonation of the noise in his body.

Both students have their legs out in front of them and their arms linked behind them. One student gently and slowly folds forward while the other gets a nice back stretch and heart opener. The students slowly come back up and then switch roles.

LIZARD SNOOZING ON A ROCK

■ **Partner Pose**

One student is in child pose. The other gently sits on her partner's back and stretches back and over the back of the student in child pose, face up like a lizard sunning itself on a rock (see figure 8.10).

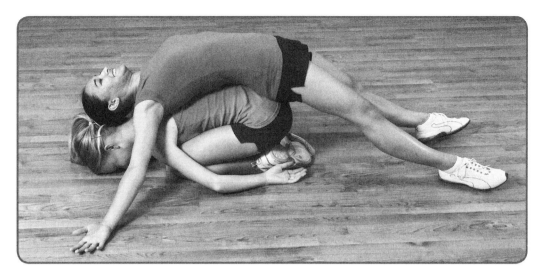

FIGURE 8.10 Lizard snoozing on a rock.

MIRROR, MIRROR

▪ **Partner Pose**

Partners face each other either sitting cross-legged, standing, or sitting back on the heels. Students place their palms against each other lightly, then hold them about 1 inch (2.5 cm) from each other. One student is the leader, and the other follows and mirrors all the movements his partner makes without talking.

PARTNER BRIDGE

▪ **Partner Pose**

Start

The students stand facing a partner. Have enough space so both partners can hinge at the hips and fold forward. The students hold onto each other's wrists or shoulders, coming into the shape of a bridge (see figure 8.11).

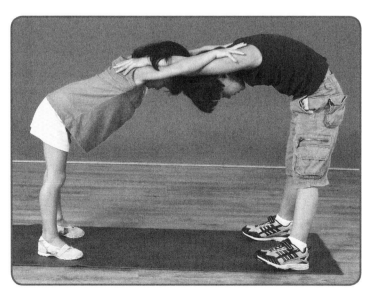

FIGURE 8.11 Partner bridge.

UPWARD-FACING BOATS

▨ Partner Pose

Students are seated and face each other. Each comes into boat pose and puts her feet against her partner's feet, holding their boat balanced. Students can hold onto each other's wrists (see figure 8.12).

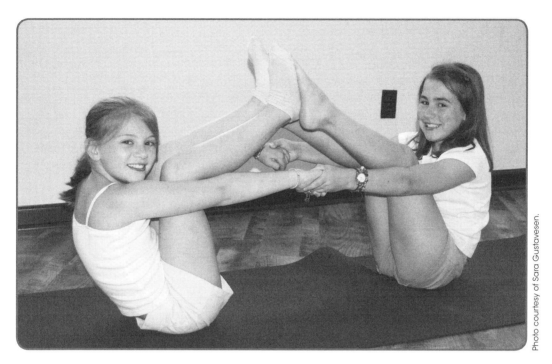

FIGURE 8.12   Upward-facing boats.

CREATIVE PROBLEM SOLVING AND YOGA

Yoga is a tremendous process that allows students to creatively solve problems. Creative problem solving is embedded in yoga teaching, as the students need to come up with the best way to make the yoga pose work for them. Included here are some ideas for exercises in creative problem solving.

Yoga sets the atmosphere for creativity and spontaneous learning by allowing students to stretch outside of their comfort zones but in a climate that is nurturing and respectful. This allows students to enjoy learning and not see physical activity as punitive, isolating, and focusing on their weaknesses but rather supportive of sharing their strengths and supporting their growth in all the challenges they face, including academics.

CROSSING THE JUNGLE RIVER

▪ **Creative Problem Solving for Younger Students**

One student "crosses the river." All the others lie facedown on the floor, as if they are floating like logs in a river, but they are really crocodiles (the students do crocodile pose). As the student makes his way around the other students, if he touches a student who is lying down, he becomes a crocodile, and the other student gets her turn to cross the river.

I ZIG AND YOU ZAG

▪ **Creative Problem Solving**

You demonstrate a pose, and the students come up with a pose that is opposite or allows the body to come into balance. For example, you do standing forward fold, and the students do a standing back bend.

NAME THAT POSE

▪ **Creative Problem Solving**

You demonstrate any yoga pose, and the students come up with a fun and different name for the yoga pose. For example, wide-angle forward fold could be "stepping out onto the ice on ice skates for the first time pose."

STRIKE A POSE

▪ **Creative Problem Solving**

You come up with a name for a pose, and the students come up with the pose (e.g., "getting a valentine from your best friend pose").

TRUST WALK

▪ **Creative Problem Solving for Older Students**

One student is blindfolded, and her partners (one or two students) guide her through obstacles by holding her elbow.

TRUSTING CIRCLE

▦ **Creative Problem Solving for Older Students**

One student stands in the middle of the circle in mountain pose, with her arms at her sides or crossed over her chest. The rest of the group stands in a circle and gently helps that person back to mountain as she falls forward, sideways, and backward with her feet glued to the floor. Now it is another student's turn (see figure 8.13).

GLOBAL AWARENESS AND YOGA

Another important part of education is cultivating responsible citizenship, civic engagement, and stewardship of this fragile earth. The exercises in this section help student realize they are an integral part of this whole world, and what they do and think influences not only their health but also the health of everyone else.

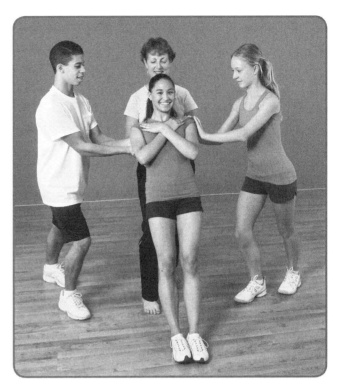

FIGURE 8.13 Trusting circle.

THINKING GLOBALLY

▦ **Global Awareness**

There are many ways that students can become more globally aware and stewards of a healthier earth. Yoga is a holistic practice that focuses on not only the physical, social, intellectual, and spiritual aspects of growth and development but the global aspects as well and how all of these are interconnected.

Brainstorm with students on ways they can start taking an active role in increasing global awareness. Have students break into groups and select one of the ideas the class came up with. Ask them to design a poster and give a persuasive presentation to the class on why that measure should be adopted. Following are some possible topics for the posters and suggestions for activities:

- Practice yoga outdoors.
- Plant a garden; learn about locally grown food and organic food.
- Invite a farmer to talk to the class so the students can learn about farming.

- Collect vegetable and fruit scraps from the cafeteria, and start a composting center.
- Clean up a neighborhood park.
- Start a fair-trade coffee and tea concession stand for the staff break room, and donate the proceeds to a green cause.
- Start recycling, and learn how to make the school greener.
- Start a green team at the school—a club that finds ways to make the school and community more earth friendly.
- Participate in National Walk to School Day.
- Volunteer at an animal shelter, or help walk the dogs.
- Have a rescue pet in the classroom to take care of.
- Find natural objects to make into art.
- Reuse water glasses or individual water bottles instead of drinking bottled water and throwing away the plastic bottles.
- Find one way each week to walk instead of using an automobile.
- Find one way each week to consume fewer throwaway items.
- Make a yoga park. Find a nature trail or outdoor area. Students design stations with laminated pictures and instructions of yoga poses for participants to try as they walk the nature path. The nature path can include exercises in noticing colors, noises, shapes, types of landscape, and wildlife. Make sure to include one station that is restful and quiet.
- Adopt a cause and make a commitment to it such as mentoring younger students; providing food, supplies, or chores to groups in need; or visiting and providing activities at a facility for older adults.

ACADEMIC AREAS AND YOGA

You can infuse academic concepts, topics, or problems to solve into your yoga sessions. These yoga exercises show students how to learn and live in a healthy way and not as an isolated activity that does not connect in meaningful ways to their lives.

There is so much learning that can take place outside the walls of a classroom. These creative learning experiences help students see beyond their own world and are lessons students will not forget. You know the academic skills and challenges of your students. Finding innovative ways to include creative learning experiences in yoga class will address the all-important concept of teaching the whole child and setting your students up for success in learning.

Art

Yoga is a beautiful activity, and having students use themselves or others as models for their art is a wonderful way to capture the beauty of yoga.

THE CHRYSALIS

▪ Art for Younger Students

Let the students spend some time researching how a caterpillar becomes a butterfly through the transformation stage called the chrysalis. This is the amazing stage when the caterpillar becomes a green cocoon and transforms into a butterfly. Instruct the students to fold a piece of paper in half and draw the same design on both sides for the wings of the butterfly. After the students have decorated their butterflies, attach a length of string and let them fly from the ceiling.

COLOR MY BREATHING

▪ Art

The students draw a picture of someone breathing in and someone breathing out. They color and shape the breath as it feels to them. Ask the students, "What color did you choose for the inhale and why? The exhale? Can you use words as well to show how breathing should feel?"

TRACE A POSE

▪ Art

On a roll of white newsprint, have students "strike a pose" such as tree or standing bow. Another student traces around the posing student. The students then color and decorate the poses.

YOGA T-SHIRT

▪ Art

Using fabric markers or paint, students put their favorite poses or statements from yoga on inexpensive white T-shirts. Examples are "Down dogs are our best friends," "Have a yoga day," and "Yoga equals peace and love" (see figure 8.14).

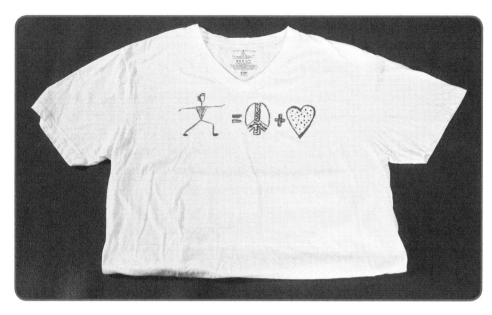

FIGURE 8.14 Yoga T-shirt.

MAKING ART FOR OTHERS

Art for Older Students

Students create art with yoga messages to give to others. Using permanent markers, the students can decorate coffee mugs, or they can design mouse pads on the computer and transfer the designs to real mouse pads. Give the class clay so they can make figurines doing yoga poses. Students can make up and illustrate yoga slogans (see figure 8.15)

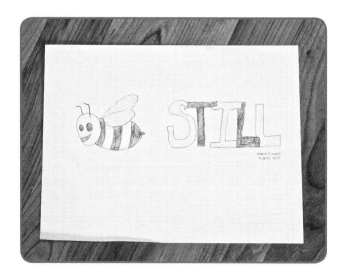

FIGURE 8.15 Yoga slogan example.

Mandalas are circular shapes that represent wholeness—they are colored vibrantly and can include symbols that are meaningful to the students, similar to a family crest. See the resource section on more ideas for including mandalas in yoga.

SHELL NECKLACE OR BRACELET AND POSES ON THE BEACH

■ Art for Older Students

Students can create a piece of shell art or jewelry and also have fun doing yoga poses that connect with going to the beach. Some of these poses include eagle (now called seagull), tree (now called palm tree), and downward-facing dog (now called crab).

Literacy

Bringing the joy of reading into your students' lives is one way you can influence them in positive ways for a lifetime. Using yoga as a means to infuse literacy is a great way to do just this.

ALPHABET SOUP AND LEARNING LETTERS

■ Literacy for Younger Students

Use various movements to mimic letters and spell out words. For X, the students can jump out into an X formed by the legs and arms; for Y, they jump the feet back together while the arms stay up; and for T, the students can do Warrior III.

MAKE UP A RHYME

■ Literacy for Younger Students

Here is an example of a sequence of yoga poses set to a rhyme for younger students.

I raise my arms and tickle the sky. (sun salutation)

And then I bend in half as I fly. (airplane arms into forward fold)

I sit right down in a comfy chair. (chair pose)

And then shoot like a rocket into the air. (rocket ship into standing up while arms reach overhead)

I can bend left, and I can bend right. (quarter moons each way)

See me cover my heart and smile bright. (mountain pose with hands over the heart space)

EVERYDAY WARRIORS

▦ **Literacy**

In yoga, the warrior is the peacekeeper. Ask the students if they can think of different attributes or characteristics of a warrior that they can use every day. Students can draw themselves doing the warrior and add words such as *courage*, *listening*, and *caring* to describe their warriors. They can decorate their warriors with different costumes.

Older students can write a story about a time they were a warrior (e.g., when they helped a friend who was in trouble or helped out in a situation that needed a strong and kind person). Find stories in the news of everyday heroes, and display them in your classroom or in a PowerPoint presentation.

I AM A MOUNTAIN

▦ **Literacy**

Ask the students to write a story or a poem about being a mountain or a tree for a day, including all the experiences that mountain or tree has that day.

STATE, NATIONAL, OR WORLD GEOGRAPHY

▦ **Literacy**

Make up movements and poses to emulate geographical landmarks and trademarks:

- What is our state tree? (tree pose)
- What is our state's largest lake? (frog pose, boat pose)
- Where is our state capital? (a motto that can be infused with a yoga pose)

RELAXATION SCRIPTS

▦ **Literacy for Older Students**

Students write their own scripts describing a relaxing place they love to visit during their relaxation time.

Books

There are many fun ways to expand your selection of books to use in yoga class. You can ask your students to bring in their favorite books, or find out what books the school is reading by asking the school librarian. Public libraries are also great resources, as most of them have a children's section with a children's literary specialist as a resource for ideas. Spending some time at a bookstore can also give you ideas, and tag sales or community book sales can be a great way to load up on books to use. Most states have a consortium or clearinghouse for children's books, or if you have a university nearby, they often let community members access their databases or can order a book for you to borrow. Ask your friends to clean out their closets of old books they may be willing to donate.

With older students, find books that have themes from yoga (such as courage, telling the truth, and nonharming) to use in a yoga class and later discuss or use in journal writing. Most electronic bookstores also have a best-seller section for younger readers where popular books can be found as well as award-winning books. Books written in other languages allow you to integrate other cultures into the yoga class. See the resource section for more ideas as well as books that come with music that can be used for a yoga class.

The following are only two examples of ways books and storytelling can be integrated with yoga for younger students by changing the names of the poses to reflect aspects of the story. For example, tree pose could be pine tree pose if the story takes place in a pine forest, or child pose could be iceberg pose if the story takes place in the cold North Pole, or it can be snail or seedling pose if the story takes place in a garden.

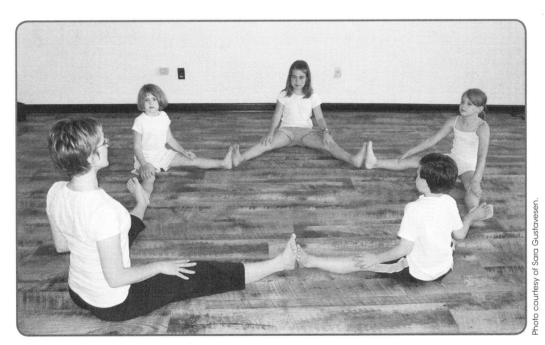

Photo courtesy of Sara Gustavesen.

Storytelling and yoga poses can be combined to help students experience a story physically.

THE BERENSTAIN BEARS ON THE MOON

▪ **Books**

A sun and moon salutation sequence of poses can be done while reading this book, such as chair (sitting in a rocket ship), rocket ship (blasting off to the moon), tipping star pose, star pose, child pose (craters), and walking on the moon (slow-motion walking or moon walking).

DR. SEUSS' *MY MANY COLORED DAYS*

▦ **Books**

This book talks about expressing emotions through color and animals. Use different poses, and ask the students to imagine coloring their poses: "Can you make your tree pose blue? Red?"

Science

Yoga poses emulate the natural world: the solar system, the cycles of the moon, animals, plants, even rocks. There is so much wisdom we can gain by observing and emulating nature, thus making learning come alive.

EXPLORING MY ENVIRONMENT

▦ **Science**

Students can infuse yoga poses as they study and capture through photos or video their exploration of the environment on a field trip or during an outdoor science lab.

THE FARM

▦ **Science**

Preschool students love poses that imitate the farm (e.g., cow or horse pose). Include discussions on why farms are important.

NATURE AND YOGA POSES

▦ **Science**

This activity relates the different poses that emulate nature, such as quarter moon, sun salute, tipping star, or side plank (can be called rainbow for this activity). Include a discussion about how we can take better care of the earth. Students can also discuss how we plant seeds to grow into a favorite plant or tree and what the plant needs in order to grow, such as rich and strong soil, sunlight, and water in balance (not too strong or hard soil or too much sun or water). This can be related to what our own bodies need for healthy and balanced living, such as good nutrition, rest, and exercise.

BRIDGE AND TRIANGLE POSES

▪ **Science for Older Students**

Using the bridge pose, ask the students to think about what makes a strong and well-designed bridge. Find examples of bridges from all over the world. Discuss the principles of design that make a strong bridge. Mathematical concepts can be brought to light using the triangle pose or standing wide-angle forward fold. Making the base of the triangle wider actually makes the structure more stable and stronger, and the students realize this through experimenting with the pose.

SUMMARY

Yoga is a gift you give your students and you give yourself as an instructor. Yoga provides an opportunity for both students and teachers to grow in healthy and balanced living as individuals and as a group. Remember that your yoga class can be the one place in a student's day that he feels good about himself and safe. Yoga is a wonderful gift for both you and your students to share. All you and your students need to do is keep the following in mind: Practice yoga and live life with an open heart and mind.

This traditional Tibetan final salutation captures how yoga is a vehicle for healthy and balanced living:

May all beings have happiness and the cause of happiness.

May all beings be free from suffering and the cause of suffering.

May all beings never be parted from freedom's true joy.

May all beings dwell in equanimity, free from attachment and aversion.

The very best to you as you bring light, energy, health, balance, and joy to your students through yoga. Namaste.

References and Resources

REFERENCES

AAHPERD. *Shape of the Nation Report.* www.aahperd. org/naspe/ShapeOfTheNation/template. cfm?template=pressRelease.html.

Alexander, K. (2002). Yoga at school poses a learning opportunity. Classroom: Teachers note calming effect, better concentration among their students. *Los Angeles Times*, 28 April 2002.

The Art of Yoga Project. www.theartofyogaproject.org/ background.php.

Bauman, A. (2002). Is yoga enough to keep you fit? www. yogajournal.com/practice/739.cfm.

Berenstain, S., & Berenstain, J. (1985). *The Berenstain Bears on the moon.* New York: Random House.

Brainy Quotes. *Albert Einstein.* www.brainyquote.com/ quotes/authors/a/albert_einstein.html

Brainy Quotes. *George Bernard Shaw.* www.brainyquote. com/quotes/quotes/g/georgebern161559.html.

Burgeson, C.R., Wechsler, H., Brener, N.D., Young, J.C., & Spain, C.G. (2001). Physical education and activity: Results from the school health policies and programs study 2000. *Journal of School Health* 71: 279-293.

Carlson, S.A., Fulton, J.E., Lee, S.M., Maynard, M., Brown, D.R., Kohl, H.W., & Dietz, W.M. (2008). Physical education and academic achievement in elementary school: Data from the early childhood longitudinal study. *American Journal of Public Health* 98(4): 721-727.

Castleman, M. (2002). Making the grade: San Francisco yoga teacher Tony Sanchez is teaching inner city students an important life skill—stress management. *Yoga Journal* (December): 91-95.

Centers for Disease Control and Prevention. *Healthy Youth.* www.cdc.gov/healthyyouth/overweight/ index.htm.

Centers for Disease Control and Prevention. *Morbidity and Mortality Weekly Report.* www.cdc.gov/mmwr/ PDF/SS/SS5505.pdf.

Children of the Night. www.childrenofthenight.org/ home.html.

Gardner, H., & Hatch, T. (1989). Multiple intelligences go to school: Educational implications of the theory of multiple intelligences. *Educational Researcher* 18(8): 4-10.

Iowa State University Extension. *Taking Charge of Stress.* www.extension.iastate.edu/publications/PM1660F. pdf.

Jensen, P.S., & Kenny, D.T., (2004). The effects of yoga on the attention and behavior of boys with attention-deficit/hyperactivity disorder (ADHD). *Journal of Attention Disorders* 7(4): 205-216.

Kassow, D. (2004). Effects of yoga on young children with or at risk for developmental disabilities or delays. *Bridges* 2(3):1-11.

Khalsa, S. K. (1998). *Fly Like A Butterfly. Yoga for Children.* New York: Sterling Publishing Co.

Kiselica, M.S., Baker, S.B., Thomas, R.N., & Reedy, S. (1994). Effects of stress inoculation training on anxiety, stress, and academic performance among adolescents. *Journal of Counseling Psychology* 41(3): 335-342.

Klimas, N. (2003, February 19). Yoga for youngsters. *Advance for Physical Therapists and PT Assistants.* http:// physical-therapy.advanceweb.com/Editorial/Search/ AViewer.aspx?CC=9200.

The Lineage Project. www.lineageproject.org.

Manjunath, N.K., & Telles, S. (2004). Spatial and verbal memory test scores following yoga and fine arts camps for school children. *Indian Journal of Physiology and Pharmacology* 48(3): 353-356.

National Association for Sport and Physical Education. (2004). *Moving into the future. National standards for physical education* (2nd ed.). Reston, VA: Author.

Norlander, T., Moas, L., & Archer, T. (2005). Noise and stress in primary and secondary school children: Noise reduction and increased concentration ability through a short but regular exercise and relaxation program. *School Effectiveness and School Improvement* 16(1): 91-99.

Palmer, P. (1997). *The courage to teach: Exploring the inner landscape of a teacher's life.* San Francisco: Jossey-Bass.

Peck, H., Kehle, T.J., Bray, M.A., & Theodore, L.E. (2005). Yoga as an intervention for children with attention problems. *School Psychology Review* 34(3): 415-424.

The Quotations Page. *Albert Einstein.* www.quotationspage.com/quote/5073.html.

Raub, J. (2002). Psychophysiologic effects of hatha yoga on musculoskeletal and cardiopulmonary function: A literature review. *Journal of Alternative and Complementary Medicine* 8(6): 797-812.

Robison, J. *Health at Every Size.* www.jonrobison.net/size.html.

Seuss, T. [Dr. Seuss]. (1996). *My many colored days.* New York: Knopf.

Slovacek, S., Tucker, S., & Pantoja, B. (2003). A study of the yoga cd program at the Accelerated School. *Program Evaluation and Research Collaborative.* www.yogaed.com/pdfs/researcharticle.pdf.

Street Yoga. www.streetyoga.org.

Stueck, M., & Gloeckner, N. (2005). Yoga for children in the mirror of science: Working spectrum and practice field of the training of relaxation with elements of yoga for children. *Early Child Development and Care* 174(4): 371-377.

Stukin, S. (2001). Om schooling: As these innovative educators have discovered, assigning yoga to kids can improve test scores and reduce disruptive behavior. *Yoga Journal* (November): 88-93, 151-153.

Sumar, S. (1998). *Yoga for the special child: A therapeutic approach for infants and children with Down syndrome, cerebral palsy, and learning disabilities.* Buckingham, Virginia: Special Yoga Publications.

Synder, M., & Chlan, L. (1999). Music therapy. In *Focus on complementary health and pain management*, ed. J.J. Fitzpatrick, 3-19. New York: Springer.

Wenig, M. (2003). *Yoga kids: Educating the whole child through yoga.* New York: Stewart, Tabori, & Chang.

RESOURCES FOR CHAPTER 3

Chair Yoga

Free Office Yoga Exercises Online offers a video of chair poses: www.soundtells.com/YogaSitting/Online/index.htm.

Visual Aids for Yoga Postures

Buckley, A. (2006). *The kids' yoga deck: 50 poses and games.* San Francisco: Chronicle Books.

Lazy Lizards Yoga offers yoga equipment designed for children: http://lazylizardyoga.com/index.html.

Music and CDs

Berkner, L (2001). *Buzz buzz.* [Audio CD]. New York: Two Tomatoes Records.

Bingo Kids (2007). *Yoga child: A peaceful place inside.* [Audio CD]. Philadelphia: Bingo Records.

Carbone, C. (2005) *Songs yoga & meditations for young yogis, children, & families!* [Audio CD]. Newport, RI: Arts-in-Celebration Recordings.

Books to Use in Yoga Class With Young Children

Eley, C., & Eley, M. (2008). *Angel bear yoga: Adventure stories.* Winston-Salem, NC: Angel Bear Yoga.

Lite, L., & Fox, K. (2007). *A boy and a turtle: A children's relaxation story to improve sleep, manage stress, anxiety, anger.* Marietta, GA: Lite Books.

Lite, L. (2004). *The goodnight caterpillar: A children's relaxation story to improve sleep, manage stress, anxiety, anger.* Marietta, GA: Lite Books.

Lite, L., & Botelho, H. (1997). *The affirmation web: A believe in yourself adventure.* Marietta, GA: Lite Books.

Penchina, S., & Hoffman, S. (2004). *I am a lovable me!* Scottsdale, AZ: 2 Imagine.

RESOURCES FOR CHAPTER 4

Books on Anatomy and Physiology

Kaminoff, L.(2007). *Yoga anatomy.* Champaign, IL: Human Kinetics.

Kirk, M., & Boon, B. (2004). *Hatha yoga illustrated.* Champaign, IL: Human Kinetics.

Wilmore, J., Costill, D., & Kenney, L. (2008). *Physiology of sport and exercise* (4th Ed.). Champaign, IL: Human Kinetics.

RESOURCES FOR CHAPTER 5

Teen Music

Lite, L. (2005). *Indigo teen dreams: Guided meditation & relaxation techniques.* Marietta, GA: Lite Books.

Soulfood. (2006). *Yoga groove.* [Audio CD]. Chanhassen, MN: Soulfood Music.

RESOURCES FOR CHAPTER 7

Resources for Moving Yoga

Rea, S. (1997). *Yoga rhythms.* [Audio CD]. Malibu, CA: Gemini Sun Records.

Rea, S. (2004). *Shakti rhythms.* [Audio CD]. Malibu, CA: Gemini Sun Records.

Yoga Zone. (1998). *Yoga zone: Music for meditation.* [Audio CD]. New York: Sony BMG.

RESOURCES FOR CHAPTER 8

Resources for PE Games

Barrett, B. (2005). *Games for the whole child.* Champaign, IL: Human Kinetics.

Burk, M.C. (2002) *Station games: Fun and imaginative PE lessons.* Champaign, IL: Human Kinetics.

Dienstmann, R. (2008). *Games for motor learning.* Champaign, IL: Human Kinetics.

LeFevre, D. (2002). *Best new games.* Champaign, IL: Human Kinetics.

PE Central offers many ideas and resources for physical education games: www.pecentral.org.

Institute of Heart Math

The Institute of HeartMath is an internationally recognized nonprofit research and education organization dedicated to heart-based living: www.heartmath.org.

Resources for Mandalas

The American heart Association offers ideas for healthy living: www.americanheart.org/presenter.jhtml?identifier=3028650.

The American Heart Association is working on a joint project with the National Football League to to help kids become active: www.whatmovesu.com/index.aspx?_vw=MAIN.

Fincher, S. (2000). *Coloring mandalas.* New York: Shambhala/Random House.

The Mandala Project is a nonprofit organization dedicated to promoting peace through art and education: www.mandalaproject.org.

Diversity

The International Association of Black Yoga Teachers provides resources for instructors of color: www.blackyogateachers.com.

Literacy

Apples4theTeacher offers free elementary language arts activities, interactive educational games, reading, writing, and book making online for kids: www.apples4theteacher.com/langarts.html.

Ideas for infusing literacy into games come from Reading Is Fundamental: www.rif.org/readingplanet/gamestation/default.mspx.

About the Author

Nanette E. Tummers, EdD, is an associate professor of health and physical education at Eastern Connecticut State University in Willimantic. She has been teaching human movement, including yoga, for 30 years. She has taught yoga to various populations, including older adults, students in afterschool programs for obese adolescents and girls at risk, women in recovery, mentally challenged adults, and athletes.

Dr. Tummers is a registered yoga teacher with Yoga Alliance and a member of the International Association of Yoga Therapists. She has been a peer reviewer of the *International Journal of Yoga Therapy*, the *Journal of Health Education*, and the *Journal of Sport and Exercise Psychology*.

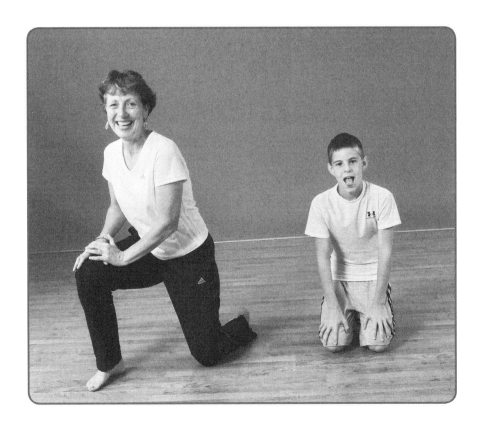

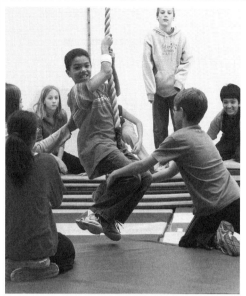
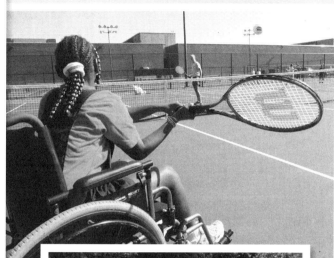
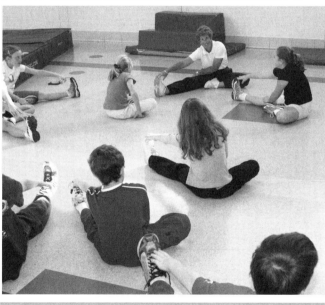
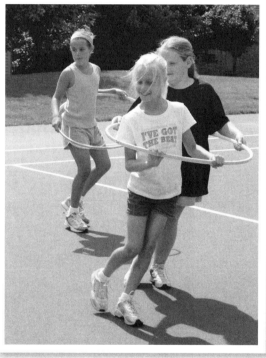

You'll find other outstanding
physical education resources at
www.HumanKinetics.com